10,000 Medical words

For Secretaries, Stenographers,
Typists, Medical Librarians,
Technicians, and Students

Compiled by Edward E. Byers, Ed.D.
Editor in Chief
Business and Management Publications
Community College Division
McGraw-Hill Book Company
New York, New York

GREGG DIVISION
McGraw-Hill Book Company
New York   St. Louis   Dallas   San Francisco
Düsseldorf   Kuala Lumpur   London   Mexico   Montreal
New Delhi   Panama   Rio de Janeiro   Singapore   Sydney   Toronto

Other Gregg/McGraw-Hill wordbooks:

10,000 Legal Words by Margaret A. Kurtz, Dorothy Adams, and Jeannette Vezeau, C.S.C.

20,000 Words, Sixth Edition, by Louis A. Leslie

Library of Congress Cataloging in Publication Data

Byers, Edward Elmer.
    10,000 medical words.

    1. Medical secretaries. 2. Medicine—Terminology.
I. Title.
R728.8.B93   610'.1'4   72-2487
ISBN 0-07-009503-5

10,000 MEDICAL WORDS

14 15 16 17 18   BKP BKP   9 0 9 8 7 6 5 4 3 2 1 0

Foreword

Medical secretaries, stenographers, typists, clerks, records librarians, technicians, nurses, and all others whose work or training for work involves the preparation of medical records and correspondence often encounter the problem of correctly spelling and dividing words not commonly used outside the medical profession. The objective of *10,000 Medical Words* is to provide the user with a convenient reference for spelling and dividing medical terms, as well as some of the more troublesome medical-related words.

THE WORD LIST

The list of more than 10,000 words and phrases in this quick reference includes many medical terms not shown in either the abridged or the unabridged editions of ordinary dictionaries. In all instances possible, however, the spelling and the syllabication of words in this reference have been checked to assure agreement with *Webster's Seventh New Collegiate Dictionary*, 1971 printing (published by G. & C. Merriam Company, Springfield, Massachusetts). The spelling and the syllabication of words not shown in that dictionary have been checked for agreement with *Webster's Third New International Dictionary* and *Dorland's Illustrated Medical Dictionary, Twenty-fourth Edition*.

Selection of Vocabulary. Because of the careful selection of the vocabulary, the list of more than 10,000 words represents the relevant part of a specialized dictionary vocabulary of several times that number. Unlike other dictionaries, this reference omits short, easily spelled words *(ill, cut)* and infrequently used or archaic words that are included in ordinary and specialized dictionaries for the sake of lexicographical completeness.

Derivative Forms. Many derivative forms are included in this reference. Frequently it is the derivative rather than the original word that is difficult to spell.

Homonyms. The medical word list contains many pairs of homonyms and words that are similar in pronunciation but different in meaning, spelling, or grammatical form—for example, *addiction* and *adduction; callous* and *callus; ileum* and *ilium.* Each pair is accompanied by very brief definitions or clues to the meaning of these words. None of these definitions or clues should be taken too literally—they are intended only to enable the reader to distinguish between two or more similar forms that might otherwise be confusing.

Compound Words. The medical word list also includes a number of words that involve the problem of whether to write them as one word, as two words, or with a hyphen. This is one of the most difficult parts of spelling. Is it *windpipe* or *wind pipe? post-natal* or *postnatal?* The answers can be found in this volume.

THE REFERENCE SECTION

The reference section that follows the medical word list contains an extensive list of medical abbreviations and acronyms. The use of medical abbreviations offers relief from the repetition of medical phrases, which can slow reading rate and obscure meaning. However, since they are subject to misinterpretation, abbreviations should be used with discretion in medical records.

Edward E. Byers

In This Book

The division of words into syllables is indicated by a centered period.

ob·ste·tri·cian   sed·i·men·ta·tion

Because the typist never breaks off a one-letter syllable at either the beginning or the end of a word, such syllables are not indicated.

*o*be·si·ty   pho·bi*a*

Syllables of two or more letters are indicated, although the typist rarely breaks off a syllable of less than three letters at the beginning or the end of a word. However, printers often break off syllables of two letters.

hy·per·acid·i·*ty*   *re*·tain·*er*

Main entries joined by the word *or* are equally acceptable.

an·hi·dro·sis *or*   ni·tro·glyc·er·in *or*
an·hy·dro·sis   ni·tro·glyc·er·ine

Homonyms and other words that are often confused are followed by a short "clue" definition and, where appropriate, *cf.* (meaning "compare").

fa·cial (pertaining to   fas·cial (pertaining to
face; cf. *fascial*)   tissue; cf. *facial*)

A

aas·mus
abac·te·ri·al
ab·alien·at·ed
ab·alien·ation
ab·ar·tic·u·la·tion
aba·sia
aba·sic
abate
abate·ment
aba·tic
ab·ax·i·al
ab·do·men
ab·dom·i·nal
ab·dom·in·al·gia
ab·dom·i·no—an·te-
ri·or
ab·dom·i·no·cen-
te·sis
ab·dom·i·no·cys·tic
ab·dom·i·no·gen·i-
tal
ab·dom·i·no·hys-
ter·ot·o·my
ab·dom·i·nos·co·py
ab·dom·i·nous
ab·dom·i·no·ves·i-
cal
ab·duce

ab·du·cent
ab·duct
ab·duc·tion
ab·duc·tor
ab·er·rant
ab·er·ra·tion (devia-
tion; cf. *abrasion*)
abey·ance
abey·ant
abi·at·ro·phy
ab·i·ent
abio·chem·is·try
abio·gen·e·sis
abio·sis
abi·ot·ro·phy
ab·ir·ri·tant
ab·ir·ri·ta·tion
ab·ir·ri·ta·tive
ab·lac·ta·tion
ablas·tin
ab·late
ab·la·tion
ableph·a·ria
ab·lu·ent
ab·lu·tion
ab·nor·mal
ab·nor·mal·i·ty
ab·oc·clu·sion
abort
abor·ti·fa·cient
abor·tion
abor·tion·ist
abor·tive
abor·tus
abrade
abra·sio

abra·sion (scraping
injury; cf. *aberration*)
abra·sive
abra·sor
ab·re·ac·tion
abro·sia
ab·scess
ab·scis·sa
ab·scis·sion
ab·sen·tia
ab·sor·be·fa·cient
ab·sor·bent
ab·sorp·tion
ab·sorp·tive
ab·ster·gent
ab·sti·nence
ab·strac·tion
abu·lia
abut·ment
abut·ted
abut·ting
aca·cia
acal·cer·o·sis
acal·ci·co·sis
acamp·sia
acan·tha
acan·thes·the·sia
acan·thoid
ac·an·tho·ma
ac·an·tho·sis
ac·an·thot·ic
acap·nia
ac·a·ri (sing.: *acarus*)
ac·a·ri·a·sis
acar·i·cide
ac·a·rid

ac·a·rus (pl.: *acari*)
acat·a·lep·sia
acat·a·lep·tic
acat·a·pha·sia
ac·a·tap·o·sis
ac·a·thex·ia
ac·cel·er·ans
ac·cel·er·a·tion
ac·cel·er·a·tor
ac·cen·tu·a·tion
ac·cep·tor
ac·ci·den·tal
ac·cli·ma·tion
ac·com·mo·da·tion
ac·couche·ment
ac·cou·cheur
ac·cou·cheuse
ac·cre·tion
acen·es·the·sia
acen·tric
ace·pha·lia
aces·o·dyne
ace·ta (sing.: *acetum*)
ac·e·tab·u·lar
ac·e·tab·u·lum
ac·et·an·i·lide *or*
   ac·et·an·i·lid
ac·et·ar·sone
ac·e·tate
ac·et·azol·amide
ace·tic
ace·ti·fy
ac·e·tim·e·ter
ac·e·tone
ac·e·to·ne·mia
ac·e·ton·uria

ac·e·to·phen·a·
   zine
ace·tous
ace·tum (pl.: *aceta*)
ace·tyl
ace·tyl·cho·line
acet·y·lene
ach·a·la·sia
ache
Achil·les
achil·lo·bur·si·tis
ach·il·lot·o·my
achlor·hy·dria
achlo·rop·sia
acho·lia
acho·lic
achor
achroi·o·cy·the·
   mia
achro·ma
achro·mach·ia
achro·ma·cyte
achro·ma·sia
ach·ro·mat
achro·ma·tin
achro·mat·o·phil
achro·ma·top·sia
achro·ma·to·sis
achro·mia
achro·mo·der·mia
Ach·ro·my·cin
achy·la·ne·mia
achy·lia
achy·lous adj.
achy·mia
acic·u·lar

ac·id
ac·i·de·mia
ac·id—fast
acid·i·fy
acid·i·ty
ac·i·do·cyte
ac·i·do·cy·to·sis
ac·i·do·phil·ic
   or ac·i·doph·
   i·lous
ac·i·do·re·sis·tant
ac·i·do·sis
acid·u·lous
ac·i·du·ria
ac·i·du·ric
ac·i·ni pl.
ac·i·nus sing.
ac·la·sis
acleis·to·car·dia
ac·mas·tic
ac·me (highest point)
ac·ne (disease)
ac·ne·form *or*
   ac·ne·iform
ac·ne·gen·ic
ac·og·no·sia
acol·o·gy
aco·mia
aco·mous adj.
ac·o·nite
acon·u·re·sis
ac·o·pro·sis
aco·rea
aco·ria
acos·mia
acou·me·ter

acou·me·try
ac·ou·o·phone
acous·ma
acous·mat·ag·no·sis
acous·ti·co·pho·bia
acous·tics
ac·ra
ac·ral
acra·sia
acra·tia
acrat·u·re·sis
ac·rid
acrit·i·cal
ac·ro—ag·no·sis
ac·ro—an·es·the·sia
ac·ro·ci·ne·sis
ac·ro·con·trac·ture
ac·ro·cy·a·no·sis
ac·ro·der·ma·ti·tis
ac·ro—ede·ma
ac·ro—es·the·sia
ac·ro·hy·po·ther·my
ac·ro·ker·a·to·sis
ac·ro·mas·ti·tis
ac·ro·meg·a·ly
ac·ro·met·a·gen·e·sis
ac·ro·mic·ria
ac·ro·mi·o·cla·vic·u·lar
acrom·pha·lus
ac·ro·my·o·to·nia

ac·ro·nym
ac·ro·nyx
ac·ro·pa·ral·y·sis
ac·ro·par·es·the·sia
ac·ro·pa·thol·o·gy
ac·rop·a·thy
ac·ro·pho·bia
ac·ro·scle·ro·sis
ac·ros·te·al·gia
acrot·ic
ac·ro·tism
ac·tin
ac·tin·o·gen
ac·tin·o·gram
ac·tin·o·graph
ac·ti·no·my·ces
ac·ti·nom·y·cin
ac·ti·nos·co·py
ac·ti·no·ther·a·py
ac·ti·va·tor
acu·ity
acu·mi·nate
ac·u·pres·sure
acu·punc·ture
acus
ac·u·sec·tion
ac·u·sec·tor
acute
acy·clia
acy·clic
ad·a·man·tine
ad·a·mas
ad·ap·ta·tion
adapt·er
ad·ax·i·al
ad·dict

ad·dic·tion (habitual use; cf. *adduction*)
ad·dic·tol·o·gist
ad·dic·tol·o·gy
ad·di·tive
ad·duct
ad·duc·tion (drawing toward; cf. *addic·tion*)
ad·duc·tor
ad·e·nal·gia
ad·en·as·the·nia
ad·e·nec·to·pia
ade·nia
ade·nic
ad·e·ni·tis
ad·e·no·blast
ad·e·no·car·ci·no·ma
ad·e·no·cele
ad·e·no·cel·lu·li·tis
ad·e·no·cys·to·ma
ad·e·no·dyn·ia
ad·e·no·fi·bro·ma sing.
ad·e·no·fi·bro·mas *or* ad·e·no·fi·bro·ma·ta pl.
ad·e·no·hy·per·sthe·nia
ad·e·noid
ad·e·noi·dal
ad·e·noid·ec·to·my
ad·e·noid·itis
ad·e·no·ma

ad·e·no·ma·la·cia
ad·e·no·ma·toid
ad·e·no·ma·tome
ad·e·no·ma·to·sis
ad·e·no·my·o·ma
ad·e·no·my·o·sis
ad·e·non·cus
ad·e·nop·a·thy
ad·e·no·phar·yn-
 gi·tis
ad·e·no·scle·ro·sis
ad·e·no·sis
ad·e·no·tome
ad·e·not·o·my
ad·e·no·ton·sil-
 lec·to·my
ad·e·nous
ad·e·no·vi·rus
ad·e·pha·gia
adeps
ad·he·sion
ad·he·si·ot·o·my
ad·he·sive·ness
adi·a·do·cho·ki-
 ne·sia
adi·a·pho·re·sis
adi·a·pho·ria
adip·ic
ad·i·po·pex·is
ad·i·pose
ad·i·po·ses pl.
ad·i·po·sis sing.
ad·i·pos·i·ty
adip·sia
ad·i·tus
ad·jec·tion

ad·junct
ad·ju·vant
ad·me·di·al or
 ad·me·di·an
ad nau·se·am
ad·nexa
ad·o·les·cence n.
ad·o·les·cent adj., n.
ad·oral
adre·nal adj.
ad·re·nal·ec·to-
 mize
ad·re·nal·ec·to·my
Adren·a·lin (trade-
 mark)
adren·a·line
ad·re·nal·ism
ad·re·na·li·tis
ad·re·nal·o·pa·thy
adro·mia
ad·sor·bent
ad·sorp·tion
adul·ter·ant
adul·ter·a·tion
ad·vance·ment
ad·ven·ti·tious
ad·vi·tant
ad·y·na·mia
aer·at·ed
aer·a·tion
ae·ri·al adj.
aer·i·al n.
aer·if·er·ous
aer·obe
aer·o·bic
aero·dy·nam·ics

aer·o·gas·tria
aer·o·gen·e·sis
aer·o·gen·ic or
 aer·og·e·nous
aer·op·a·thy
aero·pause
aer·oph·a·gy
aer·o·scope
aero·sol
aero·sol·i·za·tion
aero·ther·a·peu-
 tics
afeb·rile
af·fect
af·fer·ent (toward
 center; cf. efferent)
af·fer·en·tia
af·fin·i·ty
af·fir·ma·tion
af·flux
af·fu·sion
af·ter·birth
aga·lac·tia
agal·or·rhea
agar or agar—agar
aga·ric
agen·e·sis
ager·a·sia
ageu·sia
ag·ger
ag·glu·ti·nant
ag·glu·ti·nin
ag·gre·gate
ag·gre·ga·tion
ag·gres·sion
ag·i·tat·ed

ag·i·ta·tion
ag·i·to·pha·sia
aglo·bu·lia
aglos·sia
ag·mi·nat·ed
ag·nail
ag·nea
ag·no·sia
ag·om·phi·a·sis
agom·phi·ous
ag·o·nal
ag·o·ny
ag·o·ra·pho·bia
agrafe *or*
  agraffe
agran·u·lo·cy·to·sis
agraph·ia
agre·mia
ag·ria
agri·us
ag·ro·ma·nia
agryp·nia
ague
ail·ment
akat·a·ma·the·sia
ak·a·thi·sia
ak·i·ne·sia
akin·es·the·sia
ala sing.
alae pl.
ala·lia
alar
al·ba
al·ba·tion
al·be·do
al·bi·nism

al·bi·no
al·bu·gin·ea
al·bu·men (egg white)
al·bu·min (protein
  substance)
al·bu·mi·nate
al·bu·min·oid
al·bu·mi·no·sis
al·bu·min·ous
al·bu·min·uria
al·bu·mose
al·bu·mo·su·ria
al·co·hol
al·co·hol·e·mia
al·co·hol·ic
al·co·hol·ism
al·co·hol·om·e·ter
al·co·hol·u·ria
al·de·hyde
aleu·ke·mia
aleu·kia
aleu·ko·cy·to·sis
alex·ia
al·gae
al·ge·os·co·py
al·ge·sia
al·ge·sic
al·ge·sim·e·ter
al·ge·si·o·gen·ic
al·ges·the·sia
al·ges·the·sis
al·get·ic
al·gid
al·gin·u·re·sis
al·go·ge·ne·sia
al·go·gen·ic

al·go·lag·nia
al·go·pho·bia
al·gor
al·go·spasm
al·i·ble
alien·ation
align·ment
al·i·ment
al·i·men·ta·ry
al·i·men·ta·tion
al·i·quot
al·ka·le·mia
al·ka·li sing.
al·ka·lies *or*
  al·ka·lis pl.
al·ka·line
al·ka·lin·i·ty
al·ka·liz·er
al·ka·lo·gen·ic
al·ka·loid
al·ka·lo·sis
al·kap·ton·u·ria
  or al·cap·ton·u·
  ria
al·ler·gen
al·ler·gen·ic
al·ler·gic
al·ler·gist
al·ler·gy
al·li·ga·tion
al·lod·ro·my
al·log·a·my
al·lo·ki·ne·sis
al·lo·plas·ty
al·lo·trans·plan·
  ta·tion

5

al·loy
al·mond
alo·gia
al·o·pe·cia
al·pha
al·pho·der·mia
al·ter·e·go·ism
al·ter·nans
al·ter·nat·ing
al·tric·ious
al·um
alu·mi·na
alu·mi·num
al·ve·o·lar
al·ve·o·lec·to·my
al·ve·o·li (sing.: *alve-olus*)
al·ve·o·lo·cla·sia
al·ve·o·lo·plas·ty
al·ve·o·lot·o·my
al·ve·o·lus (pl.: *alve-oli*)
al·ve·us (canal; cf. *alvus*)
al·vi (sing.: *alvus*)
al·vi·no·lith
al·vus (pl.: *alvi;* abdomen; cf. *alveus*)
alym·phia
al·ys·o·sis
am·a·tho·pho·bia
am·a·tive·ness
am·a·to·ry
am·au·ro·ses pl.
am·au·ro·sis sing.
am·au·rot·ic

amax·o·pho·bia
am·ber·gris
am·bi·dex·ter·i·ty
am·bi·dex·trous
am·bi·le·vous
am·bi·oc·u·lar·i·ty
am·biv·a·lence
am·bi·vert
am·bly·o·pia
am·bu·lance
am·bu·lant
am·bu·la·to·ry
am·bus·tion
am·e·bi·a·sis
ame·bic
am·el·e·ia
amen·or·rhea
amim·ia
am·mo·nia
am·mo·nium
am·ne·mon·ic
am·ne·sia
am·ni·on
amoe·ba sing.
amoe·bas *or* amoe·bae pl.
amoe·boid
amok
amor·phous
amo·ti·o·ret·i·nae
am·phi·ar·thro·sis
am·phi·chro·ic
am·phi·cra·nia
am·phig·o·ny
am·phor·ic
am·pho·ric·i·ty

am·pho·ril·o·quy
am·pli·fi·ca·tion
am·poule *or* am·pul
am·pul·la sing.
am·pul·lae pl.
am·pu·tate
am·pu·ta·tion
am·pu·tee
amu·sia
am·y·dri·a·sis
am·yl
am·y·lase
am·y·loid
am·y·loi·do·sis
am·y·lon
am·y·lu·ria
Am·y·tal
ana·bi·ot·ic
anab·o·lism
an·a·cu·sis
an·a·dip·sia
an·a·lep·tic
an·al·ge·sia
an·al·ge·sic
an·al·ler·gic
anal·y·ses pl.
anal·y·sis sing.
an·a·lyst
an·a·lyt·ic
an·a·lyz·er
an·am·ne·sis
an·a·mor·pho·sis
an·an·a·ba·sia
an·an·dria
an·an·gi·o·pla·sia

6

an·a·pau·sis
an·a·pho·re·sis
anas·ta·sis
anas·to·mo·sis
anat·o·mist
anat·o·my
an·a·tox·in
an·co·ne·us
an·dro·gen
an·dro·gen·e·sis
an·droid
an·dro·pho·bia
ane·mia
an·er·gy
an·es·the·sia
an·es·the·si·ol·o·gist
an·es·the·si·ol·o·gy
an·es·thet·ic
anes·the·tist
anes·the·tize
anes·tri pl.
an·es·trous adj.
an·es·trus sing.
an·e·to·der·ma
aneu·ria
an·eu·rysm
an·gi·i·tis
an·gi·na
an·gi·o·car·di·o·gram
an·gi·o·der·ma·ti·tis
an·gi·og·ra·phy
an·gi·oid
an·gi·o·lith

an·gi·o·lith·ic
an·gi·o·ma
an·gi·op·a·thy
an·gi·or·rex·is
an·gi·o·scle·ro·sis
an·gi·o·stax·is
an·gi·os·te·o·sis
an·gi·os·to·my
an·gle
an·gor
an·gu·la·tion
an·hem·a·to·poi·e·sis
an·he·mo·lyt·ic
an·hi·dro·sis or
    an·hy·dro·sis
an·i·line
anil·i·ty
an·i·ma
an·i·mas·tic
an·i·mus
an·ise
an·iso·co·ria
an·i·so·dont
an·kle
an·ky·lo·glos·sia
an·ky·losed
an·ky·lo·sis
an·la·ge sing.
an·la·gen pl.
an·neal
an·nec·tent
an·nu·late
an·nu·li pl.
an·nu·lo·sa
an·nu·lose adj.

an·nu·lus sing.
an·ode
an·o·don·tia
an·o·don·tous
an·o·dyn·ia
an·o·et·ic
anom·a·ly
ano·mia
an·o·op·sia or
    anop·sia
ano·plas·ty
an·orex·ia
ano·scope
an·os·mia
an·os·to·sis
an·ox·emia
an·ox·ia
an·sa sing.
an·sae pl.
ant·ac·id
an·tag·o·nism
an·tag·o·nist
an·tag·o·nize
ant·al·ka·line
an·te—ci·bum
an·te·flex·ion
an·te·mor·tem
an·te·na·tal
an·te·par·tum
an·te·ri·or
an·ter·o·dor·sal
an·te·ver·sion
an·thra·ces pl.
an·thrax sing.
an·thro·pol·o·gy
an·ti·ar·thrit·ic

an·ti·bac·ter·i·al
an·ti·bi·o·sis
an·ti·bi·ot·ic
an·ti·body
an·ti·car·i·ous
an·ti·co·ag·u·lant
an·ti·com·ple·ment
an·ti·con·vul·sive
an·ti·di·a·bet·ic
an·ti·dot·al
an·ti·dote
an·ti·fe·brile
an·ti·gen
an·ti·gen·ic
an·ti·ge·nic·i·ty
an·ti·hem·or·rhoid·al
an·ti·his·ta·mine
an·ti·sep·sis
an·ti·sep·tic
an·ti·se·rum
an·ti·tox·in
an·ti·ven·in
an·tra pl.
an·trum sing.
an·ure·sis
an·uria
anus
anx·i·ety
aor·ta
aor·tal
aor·tic
ap·a·thy
ap·er·tu·ra
ap·er·ture
apex sing.

apex·es or api·ces pl.
apha·gia
apha·sia
apheix·ia
apho·nia
aph·tha sing.
aph·thae pl.
apla·sia
aplas·tic
ap·nea or ap·noea
apo·neu·ro·sis
apoph·y·sis
ap·o·plexy
apos·ta·sis
ap·pa·ra·tus
ap·pend·age
ap·pen·dec·to·my
ap·pen·di·cec·to·my
ap·pen·di·ci·tis
ap·pen·dix
ap·per·cep·tion
ap·pe·tite
ap·pe·tiz·er
ap·pli·ca·tor
ap·po·si·tion
ap·prox·i·mal
aprax·ia
apty·a·lism
apy·rex·ia
aq·ua sing.
aq·uae or aq·uas pl.
arach·noid
arach·noid·i·tis
ar·cade
ar·cha·ic

ar·che·type
ar·ci·form
ar·cu·a·tion
ar·cus
are·o·la sing.
are·o·lae or are·o·las pl.
are·o·lar
arm·pit
ar·o·mat·ic
ar·rest
ar·rhyth·mia
ars·a·man·di
ar·se·nic
ar·te·ri·o·gram
ar·te·ri·og·ra·phy
ar·te·ri·ole
ar·te·ri·o·lith
ar·te·ri·o·ma·la·cia
ar·te·ri·or·rha·phy
ar·te·ri·or·rhex·is
ar·te·rio·scle·ro·sis
ar·te·ri·o·ste·no·sis
ar·te·ri·o·tome
ar·te·ri·ot·o·my
ar·te·ri·tis
ar·te·ry
ar·thral·gia
ar·threc·to·my
ar·thre·de·ma
ar·thri·tis
ar·thro·cele
ar·throd·e·sis
ar·thro·lith
ar·throl·o·gy
ar·throl·y·sis

ar·throp·a·thy
ar·thro·plas·ty
ar·thro·sis
ar·thros·to·my
ar·throt·o·my
ar·tic·u·lar
ar·tic·u·late
ar·tic·u·lat·ing
ar·tic·u·la·ti·o sing.
ar·tic·u·la·ti·o-
  nes pl.
ar·tic·u·la·tion
ar·tic·u·lus
ar·ti·fi·cial
asar·cia
as·cend·ing
as·ci·tes
asep·sis
asep·tic
asex·u·al
aso·nia
as·per·ous
as·phyx·ia
as·phyx·i·ant
as·phyx·i·a·tion
as·pi·ra·tion
as·pi·ra·tor
as·pi·rin
as·say
as·sim·i·la·tion
as·so·ci·a·tion
asta·sia
as·the·nia
as·then·ic
asth·ma
astig·ma·tism

astig·mo·scope
as·trag·a·li pl.
as·trag·a·lus sing.
as·tra·pho·bia
as·trin·gent
as·tro·blas·to·ma
as·tro·cy·to·ma
asy·lum
asym·met·ric
asym·met·ri·cal
asym·me·try
asymp·tom·at·ic
asyn·er·gy
asys·tem·at·ic
atac·tic
at·a·rac·tic or
  at·a·rax·ic
atax·a·pha·sia or
  atax·i·apha·sia
atax·ia
at·e·lec·ta·sis
ath·er·o·ma
ath·e·to·sis
at·om
atom·ic
at·om·iza·tion
atox·ic
atre·mia
atre·sia
atri·um
at·ro·pho·der·ma
at·ro·phy
at·ro·pine
at·ten·u·a·tion
at·ti·tude
at·tri·tion

atyp·i·cal
au·di·o·gen·ic
au·dio·vi·su·al
au·di·tion
au·di·tive
au·di·to·ry
aug·ment
aug·men·ta·tion
aug·men·tor
au·ra sing.
au·ral (of ear; cf. oral)
au·ras pl.
au·ri·cle
au·ris
au·rist
aus·cul·ta·tion
au·tism
au·tis·tic
au·to·clave
au·tom·a·tism
au·tom·a·ton
au·to·nom·ic
au·ton·o·mous
au·top·a·thy
au·top·sy
au·to·some
aux·e·sis
aux·et·ic
av·oir·du·pois
avul·sion
ax·es (sing.: axis)
ax·il·la sing.
ax·il·lae or ax-
  il·las pl.
ax·is (pl.: axes)
azure

9

B

ba·cil·la·ry
ba·cil·li pl.
ba·cil·li·form
ba·cil·lus sing.
back·ache
back·bone
back·ward·ness
bac·te·ria (sing.: bac-
    terium)
bac·te·ri·al
bac·te·ri·oid
bac·te·ri·ol·o·gist
bac·te·ri·ol·o·gy
bac·te·ri·os·co·py
bac·te·rio·sta·sis
bac·te·ri·um (pl.:
    bacteria)
baf·fle
bal·ance
bal·a·nism
bal·a·ni·tis
bal·a·nus
bal·lism or bal-
    lis·mus
bal·loon·ing
bal·lotte·ment
bal·sam
ban·dage
bar·bi·tal
bar·bi·tu·rate

bar·bi·tu·rism
bar·bo·tage
bar·es·the·sia
bar·i·um
bar·og·no·sis
ba·rom·e·ter
bar·o·tal·gia
bar·o·ti·tis
bar·ri·er
bar·y·la·lia
bar·y·pho·nia
bas·al met·a-
    bol·ic
ba·si·fa·cial
ba·si·lat·er·al
ba·sil·ic
ba·so·phil or ba-
    so·phile
ba·so·phil·ia
ba·so·phil·ic
ba·so·pho·bia
bas·si·net
bath·es·the·sia
bath·o·pho·bia
bat·tery
bed·pan
bed·rid·den or
    bed·rid
bed·sore
bel·la·don·na
bel·ly·ache
be·nign
Ben·ze·drine
ben·zene
ben·zo·caine
ben·zo·in

ben·zo·yl
ben·zyl
beri·beri
be·ta
bi·ax·i·al
bi·car·bon·ate
bi·ceps
bi·cus·pid
bi·fid
bi·fo·cal
bi·fur·ca·tion
bi·gem·i·nal
bi·gem·i·ny
bi·lat·er·al
bile (liver secretion; cf.
    bowel)
bil·i·ary
bil·ious
bi·li·ru·bin
bil·i·ru·bi·ne·mia
    or bil·i·ru·nae-
    mia
bil·i·u·ria
bi·man·u·al
bi·na·ry
bi·na·sal
bin·au·ral
bio·chem·is·try
bio·gen·e·sis
bi·o·ki·net·ics
bi·ol·o·gist
bi·ol·o·gy
bio·phys·ics
bi·op·la·sis
bi·op·sy
bio·type

bi·pa·ri·e·tal
bi·po·ten·ti·al·i·ty
birth·mark
birth·rate
bis·fe·ri·ous
bi·sex·u·al
bis·muth
bis·tou·ry
black·head
black out v.
black·out n.
blad·der
blas·te·ma sing.
blas·te·mas or
  blas·te·ma·ta pl.
blas·to·coel or
  blas·to·coele
blas·to·cyst
blas·to·derm
blas·to·gen·e·sis
blas·to·ma
blas·to·my·co·sis
blas·tu·la sing.
blas·tu·las or
  blas·tu·lae pl.
bleed·er
bleed·ing
blen·nor·rha·gia
blen·nor·rhea
bleph·a·ral
bleph·a·rit·i·des pl.
bleph·a·ri·tis sing.
bleph·a·ron
bleph·a·roph·ry-
  plas·ty
bleph·a·ro·ple·gia

bleph·a·rop·to·sis
bleph·a·ro·spasm
bleph·a·ro·stat
bleph·a·rot·o·my
bleph·so·path·ia
blind·ness
blis·ter
blood pres·sure
blood·stream
boil
bo·lus
bo·rate
bo·rax
bo·ric ac·id
bor·rel·ia
bot·a·ny
both·ri·oid
bot·u·lism
bou·gie
bouil·lon
bour·donne·ment
bow·el (intestine; cf.
  bile)
bow·legged
bra·chia (sing.:
  brachium)
bra·chi·al
bra·chi·al·gia
brach·i·al·is
bra·chi·ot·o·my
bra·chi·um (pl.:
  brachia)
brach·y·sta·sis
brady·car·dia (slow
  heartbeat; cf. tachy-
  cardia)

brad·y·crot·ic
brad·y·lex·ia
brad·y·pha·sia
brad·y·pnea
brad·y·prax·ia
brad·y·rhyth·mia
bri·dle
bro·mate
bro·mat·ed
bro·mide
bronch·ad·e·ni·tis
bron·chi (sing.: bron-
  chus)
bron·chia (sing.:
  bronchium)
bron·chi·ec·ta·sis
bron·chi·ole
bron·chit·i·des pl.
bron·chi·tis sing.
bron·chi·um (pl.:
  bronchia)
bron·cho·cele
bron·cho·con-
  stric·tor
bron·cho·dil·a·ta-
  tion
bron·cho·di·la·tor
bron·cho·e·de·ma
bron·cho·gen·ic
bron·cho·gram
bron·chog·ra·phy
bron·chol·o·gy
bron·cho·pneu·mo-
  nia
bron·cho·pul·mo-
  na·ry

bron·cho·scope
bron·chos·to·my
bron·chot·o·my
bron·chus (pl.: *bron-chi*)
bruxo·ma·nia
bryg·mus
bu·bo sing.
bu·boes pl.
bu·bon·al·gia
bu·bon·o·cele
buc·ca
buc·co—ax·i·al
buc·co·cer·vi·cal
buc·co·dis·tal
buc·co·gin·gi·val
buc·cu·la
bul·bar
bul·bous
bu·le·sis
bu·lim·ia
bul·la sing.
bul·lae pl.
bul·late
bun·ion·ec·to·my
bu·no·dont
bu·rette *or* bu·ret
bur·nish·er
bur·sa sing.
bur·sas *or* bur-sae pl.
bur·sec·to·my
bur·si·tis
bu·tane
but·tock
bu·tyl

ca·chex·ia
cach·in·na·tion
ca·chou
ca·dav·er·ous
cad·mi·um
ca·du·cei pl.
ca·du·ce·us sing.
ca·du·cous
cal·a·mine
cal·ca·ne·o·val·gus
cal·ca·ne·us
cal·car sing.
cal·car·e·ous
cal·car·ia pl.
cal·ci·fi·ca·tion
cal·ci·grade
cal·ci·pe·nia
cal·ci·um
cal·cu·li pl.
cal·cu·lus sing.
cal·e·fa·cient
cal·i·bra·tion
cal·i·bra·tor
cal·i·pers *or* cal·li·pers
cal·is·then·ics
cal·los·i·ty
cal·lous adj. (hard)
cal·lus n. (thickened skin)

cal·or
ca·lo·ric
cal·o·rie
ca·lor·i·gen·ic
cal·var·ia pl.
cal·var·i·um sing.
cal·vi·ties
cal·vous
ca·lyx sing.
ca·lyx·es *or* ca·ly·ces pl.
cam·era
cam·i·sole
cam·phor
ca·nal
can·a·lic·u·li pl.
can·a·lic·u·lus sing.
ca·nal·iza·tion
can·cel·lous
can·cer
can·cer·o·gen
can·cer·ol·o·gy
can·cer·ous
ca·nine
ca·ni·ti·es
can·ker
can·nu·la sing.
can·nu·las *or* can-nu·lae pl.
ca·pac·i·ty
cap·il·lar·ec·ta·sia
cap·il·lary
ca·pil·lus
cap·i·ta·tum
cap·i·tel·lum
ca·pit·u·la pl.

ca·pit·u·lum sing.
cap·sule
ca·put
car·ba·sus
car·bi·nol
car·bo·hy·drate
car·bol·ic ac·id
car·bon
car·bon·at·ed
car·bun·cle (inflammation with pus; cf. *caruncle, furuncle*)
car·ci·noid
car·ci·no·ma sing:
car·ci·no·mas *or* car·ci·no·ma·ta pl.
car·ci·no·ma·to·sis
car·di·ac
car·di·al·gia
car·di·ec·ta·sis
car·dio·gram
car·dio·graph
car·di·ol·o·gist
car·di·ol·o·gy
car·dio·path
car·di·o·ple·gia
car·di·o·pneu·mat·ic
car·dio·pul·mo·nary
car·dio·re·spi·ra·to·ry
car·di·or·rha·phy
car·dio·spasm
car·di·o·ste·no·sis

car·di·o·ther·a·py
car·di·ot·o·my
car·dio·vas·cu·lar
car·dio·vas·cu·lar—re·nal
car·di·tis
car·ies
car·i·ous
ca·rot·ic
ca·rot·id
ca·rot·is
car·pal
car·pus (wrist; cf. *corpus*)
car·ri·er
car·ti·lage
car·un·cle (fleshy eminence; cf. *carbuncle, furuncle*)
cas·cara
ca·se·ate
ca·se·ation
ca·se·ous
cas·sette
cas·trate
cas·tra·tion
ca·su·al·ty
ca·su·is·tic
ca·tab·a·sis
ca·tab·o·lism
cat·a·lep·sy
cat·a·lyst
cat·a·lyz·er
cat·a·pha·sia
ca·taph·o·ra
cat·a·pla·sia

cat·a·plasm
cat·a·plexy
cat·a·ract
ca·tarrh
cat·a·stal·sis
cat·gut
ca·thar·ses pl.
ca·thar·sis sing.
ca·thar·tic
ca·ther·e·sis
cath·e·ret·ic
cath·e·ter
cath·e·ter·ism
cath·ode
ca·thod·ic
cau·dad
cau·sal·gia
caus·tic
cau·ter·ant
cau·ter·i·za·tion
cau·ter·ize
cau·tery
cav·ern·ous
cav·i·tas
cav·i·ta·tion
cav·i·ty
ce·ca (sing.: *cecum* or *caecum*)
ce·co·cele
ce·cot·o·my
ce·cum *or* cae·cum (pl.: *ceca*)
ce·li·ac
ce·li·os·co·py
ce·li·ot·o·my
ce·li·tis

cel·la
cel·lu·li·tis
cel·lu·lose
ce·men·ta pl.
ce·men·tum sing.
ce·nes·the·sia
cen·te·ses pl.
cen·te·sis sing.
cen·ti·grade
cen·ti·gram
cen·ti·me·ter
cen·tri·fuge
cen·trum sing.
cen·trums or cen·tra pl.
ceph·a·lal·gia
ce·phal·ic
ceph·a·lo·cele
ceph·a·loid
ce·rate
cer·e·bel·lo·spi·nal
cer·e·bel·lum
ce·re·bral
cer·e·bra·tion
ce·re·bro·spi·nal
ce·re·brum
ce·re·ous
cer·e·sin
ce·ri·um
ce·ru·men
ce·ru·mi·no·sis
cer·vi·cal adj. (of neck or cervix; cf. *clavicle*)
cer·vi·ces (sing.: *cervix*)

cer·vi·ci·tis
cer·vi·co·ves·i·cal
cer·vix (pl.: *cervices*; neck of uterus; cf. *pelvis*)
ce·sar·e·an or ce·sar·i·an
chaf·ing
chan·cre
chapped
char·la·tan
char·ley horse
char·ta sing.
char·tae pl.
char·tu·la
check·up n.
cheek·bone
chei·li·tis or chi·li·tis
chei·lo·sis
chem·i·cal
chem·ist
chem·is·try
chem·o·sur·gery
chig·ger
chil·blain
chi·rag·ra
chi·rap·sia
chi·ris·mus
chi·rol·o·gy
chlo·rine
chlo·ro·form
chlo·ro·phyll
chok·ing
chol·an·gi·og·ra·phy

chol·an·gi·o·ma
chol·an·gi·ot·o·my
chol·an·gi·tis
cho·late
chol·e·bil·i·ru·bin
cho·le·cyst
chol·e·cyst·al·gia
chol·e·cyst·ec·ta·sia
cho·le·cys·tic
cho·le·cys·ti·tis
cho·le·cys·to·gram
chol·e·cys·to·pexy
chol·e·cys·tot·o·my
cho·led·o·chi·tis
cho·led·o·cho·li·thot·o·my
cho·led·o·chos·to·my
cho·le·glo·bin
cho·le·ic
cho·le·lith
cho·le·mia or cho·lae·mia
chol·era
cho·le·re·sis
chol·er·rha·gia
cho·les·ter·ol
cho·line
cho·lin·er·gic
cho·lin·es·ter·ase
chol·o·chrome
chol·o·lith
chol·uria

14

chon·dral
chon·drec·to·my
chon·dri·tis
chon·dro·blast
chon·dro·cos·tal
chon·dro·dys-
    tro·phia
chon·drog·e·nous
chon·dro·ma
chon·dro·ma·la·cia
chon·dro·mere
chon·drop·a·thy
chon·dro·sar·co·ma
chon·dro·sis
chon·dro·tome
chor·da
chor·di·tis
chor·do·ma
chor·dot·o·my or
    cor·dot·o·my
cho·rea
cho·ri·o·cele
cho·ri·on
cho·roid
cho·roid·itis or
    cho·ri·oid·itis
chro·mate
chro·ma·tid
chro·ma·tin
chro·ma·to·dys·o-
    pia
chro·ma·tog·ra·phy
chro·ma·tom·e·ter
chro·ma·tom·e·try
chro·ma·top·a·thy
chro·mato·phore

chro·ma·to·sis
chro·mi·um
chro·mo·cyte
chro·mo·phobe
chro·mo·pho·bic
chro·mo·plasm
chro·mos·co·py
chro·mo·some
chro·nax·ie
chyle
chy·le·mia
chy·li·dro·sis
chy·lu·ria
chyme
cil·ia (sing.: *cilium*)
cil·i·ary
cil·i·ate or
    cil·i·at·ed
cil·i·um (pl.: *cilia*)
cil·lo·sis
cin·cho·na
ci·ne·rea
cin·gu·la pl.
cin·gu·lum sing.
cin·na·mon
cir·cu·la·tion
cir·cu·la·to·ry
cir·cum·ci·sion
cir·cum·flex
cir·cum·scribe
cir·cum·stan·ti-
    al·i·ty
cir·cum·vas·cu·lar
cir·rho·sis (disease of
    liver; cf. *serosa*,
    xerosis)

cir·sec·to·my
cir·soid
cis·tern
cis·ter·na sing.
cis·ter·nae pl.
ci·trate
cit·rine
cit·ro·nel·la
clap·ping
cla·rif·i·cant
clar·i·fi·ca·tion
clas·tic
clau·di·ca·tion
claus·tro·phil·ia
claus·tro·pho·bia
cla·va (sing.: *clavus*)
cla·vate
clav·i·cle (collar bone;
    cf. *cervical*)
cla·vic·u·late
cla·vus (pl.: *clava*)
clear·ance
cleav·age
clei·do·cos·tal
cle·oid
cli·mac·ter·ic
cli·mate
clin·ic
clin·i·cal
cli·ni·cian
clit·o·ri·di·tis
cli·to·ris
clit·o·ri·tis
clit·or·rha·gia
cli·vi pl.
cli·vus sing.

clo·a·ca sing.
clo·a·cae pl.
clo·nic
clo·nus
clos·trid·i·a pl.
clos·trid·i·um sing.
clo·sure
clot·ting
club·foot
clu·ne·al
clut·ter·ing
cly·sis
cnem·i·des pl.
cne·mis sing.
co·ag·u·la (sing.: *co-agulum*)
co·ag·u·lant
co·ag·u·la·tion
co·ag·u·lum (pl.: *co-agula*)
co·ales·cence
co·ap·ta·tion
co·arc·tate
co·arc·ta·tion
co·ar·tic·u·la·tion
co·balt
co·caine
co·cain·ism
coc·ci pl.
coc·cus sing.
coc·cy·ges (sing.: *coccyx*)
coc·cyg·e·us
coc·cyx (pl.: *coc-cyges*)
coch·lea

coch·le·ar
co·deine
cod·liv·er
co·ef·fi·cient
co·en·zyme
cog·ni·tion
co·hab·i·ta·tion
co·her·ence
co·he·sion
co·i·to·pho·bia
co·itus
co·la·tion
cold sore
co·le·o·cele
co·le·op·to·sis
co·les
co·li·ba·cil·lus
col·ic n. (pain)
col·ic adj. (of colon)
col·icky
co·li·form
co·li·tis
col·lapse
col·lar·bone
col·lat·er·al
col·lic·u·lus
col·lin·ear
col·li·sion
col·lo·di·on
col·loid
col·loi·dal
col·lum
col·lu·nar·i·um
col·lyr·ia *or* col·lyr·i·ums pl.
col·lyr·i·um sing.

col·o·bo·ma
col·o·cynth
co·lon
co·lop·to·sis
col·or
co·los·to·my
co·los·tror·rhea
co·los·trum
col·pal·gia
col·pec·ta·sia
col·pe·de·ma
col·pi·tis
col·po·pexy
col·po·scope
col·umn
co·lum·na sing.
co·lum·nae pl.
co·ma
co·ma·tose
comb·ing
com·e·do sing.
com·e·do·nes pl.
co·mes
com·mi·nute
com·mis·su·ra
com·mis·sure
com·mo·tio
com·mu·ni·ca·ble
com·mu·ni·ca·tion
com·pat·i·bil·i·ty
com·pen·sa·tion
com·pen·sa·to·ry
com·pe·tence
com·ple·ment
com·ple·men·tal
com·ple·men·ta·ry

16

com·plex
com·plex·ion
com·pli·ca·tion
com·po·nent
com·po·si·tion
com·pound
com·press
com·pres·sion
com·pres·sor
com·pul·sion
com·pul·sive
co·na·tion
con·cave
con·ceive
con·cen·tra·tion
con·cen·tric
con·cep·tion
con·cep·tus
con·cha
con·com·i·tant
con·cre·ment
con·cres·cence
con·cre·tion
con·cus·sion (jar or shock; cf. *contusion, convulsion*)
con·den·sa·tion
con·dens·er
con·di·tion·ing
con·duct·ibil·i·ty
con·duc·tion
con·dyle
con·dy·lo·ma
con·fab·u·la·tion
con·fec·tion
con·fer·tus

con·fine·ment
con·flu·ence
con·flu·ent
con·fu·sion
con·ge·la·tion
con·gen·i·tal
con·ges·tion
con·glo·bate
con·glom·er·ate
con·glu·ti·nant
con·i·cal
con·i·za·tion
con·ju·gate
con·ju·ga·tion
con·junc·ti·va sing.
con·junc·ti·vas *or* con·junc·ti·vae pl.
con·junc·ti·vi·tis
co·noid
con·san·guin·e·ous
con·san·guin·i·ty
con·scious·ness
con·sis·tence
con·sis·ten·cy
con·sol·i·dant
con·sper·gent
con·stant
con·stel·la·tion
con·sti·pa·tion
con·sti·tu·tion
con·stric·tor
con·sul·tant
con·sul·ta·tion
con·sump·tion
con·tact

con·ta·gion
con·tam·i·nant
con·tam·i·nate
con·tam·i·nat·ing
con·tam·i·na·tion
con·tem·plate
con·tem·pla·tive
con·tig·u·ous
con·ti·nence
con·tin·gen·cy
con·tor·tion
con·tour
con·tra·cep·tion
con·tra·cep·tive
con·trac·til·i·ty
con·trac·tion
con·trac·ture
con·tra·stim·u·lant
con·tre·coup
con·trude
con·tu·sion (bruise; cf. *concussion, convulsion*)
co·nus
con·va·les·cence n.
con·va·les·cent adj., n.
con·vec·tion
con·vex·i·ty
con·vexo—con·cave
con·vo·lu·tion
con·vul·sion (contraction of muscles; cf. *concussion, contusion*)

co·or·di·na·tion
cop·i·o·pia
cop·ro·lith
cop·u·la·tion
cor·dial
cor·ec·ta·sis
cor·ec·tome
cor·e·om·e·ter
co·re·ste·no·ma
cor·nea
cor·ne·ous
cor·nu sing.
cor·nua pl.
co·ro·na
cor·o·na·le
cor·o·nary
cor·o·ner (person)
cor·po·ra (sing.: *cor·pus*)
corpse
cor·pus (pl.: *corpora;* main body; cf. *car·pus*)
cor·pus·cle
cor·pus·cu·lar
cor·pus·cu·lum
cor·pus de·lic·ti
cor·rec·tive
cor·re·la·tion
cor·re·spon·dence
cor·ro·sion
cor·ru·ga·tor
cor·set
cor·tex sing.
cor·ti·ces or cor·tex·es pl.

cor·ti·co·troph·in or cor·ti·co·tro·pin
cor·ti·sone
cor·us·ca·tion
co·ry·za
cos·met·ic
cos·ta
cos·tal·gia
cos·tal·is
cos·tec·to·my
cos·tive
cos·to·chon·dral
cos·to·tome
cos·to·ver·te·bral
cot·ton
cough
coun·ter·ac·tion
co·va·lence or co·va·len·cy
coxa sing.
cox·ae pl.
cox·al·gia
cox·i·tis
cra·dle
cra·ni·al
cra·ni·ol·o·gy
cra·ni·um
cran·ter
crap·u·lent
cre·mate
cre·ma·tion
cre·ma·to·ry
cre·o·sote
crep·i·tant
crep·i·ta·tion
cres·cent

cre·ta
cre·tin·ism
crev·ice
crib·bing
crib·ri·form
crick
cri·coid
cri·no·sin
cri·ses pl.
cri·sis sing.
cris·ta
crit·i·cal
crossed
cross·ing—over
crotch
croup
croupy
crutch
crypt
crys·tal·line
crys·tal·li·za·tion
cu·bi·ti pl.
cu·bi·tus sing.
cul—de—sac
cu·li·cide
cul·men
cul·ture
cu·ne·i·form
cun·nus
cupped
cur·age (of a cure)
cu·ra·tive
cu·ret·tage
cu·rette or cu·ret
cur·rent
cur·va·ture

cus·pid
cu·ta·ne·ous
cu·ti·cle
cu·tic·u·la
cu·tis *or*
  cu·tis ve·ra .
cy·an·a·mide
cy·a·nide
cy·a·no·sis
cy·a·not·ic
cy·ber·net·ics
cy·cla·mate
cy·cle
cy·clic
cy·cloid
cy·clo·tron
cy·e·si·og·no·sis
cy·e·sis
cyl·in·der
cy·lin·dri·form
cyl·in·dro·ma
cyl·lo·sis
cy·no·bex
cy·o·pho·ria
cyst·ad·e·no·ma
cys·tal·gia
cyst·ec·ta·sia
cys·tec·to·my
cys·tic
cys·ti·tis
cys·to·car·pic
cys·to·cele
cys·to·gram
cys·toid
cys·to·ma
cys·to·pexy

cys·to·scope
cys·tos·co·py
cys·tos·to·my
cys·to·tome
cy·to·blast
cy·to·cide
cy·toc·la·sis
cy·tode
cy·to·gen·e·sis
cy·tol·o·gy
cy·tom·e·ter
cy·ton
cy·to·phil
cy·to·plasm
cy·to·some

dac·tyl
dac·ty·li·tis
dac·tyl·o·gram
dac·ty·lo·meg·a·ly
dac·ty·lus
dan·druff
de·ac·ti·va·tion
deaf·ness
de·al·ler·gi·za·tion
de·bil·i·tant
de·bil·i·ty
de·bride·ment

de·bris
de·cal·ci·fi·ca·tion
deca·li·ter
deca·me·ter
de·cant
de·car·bon·ate
de·cay
de·cel·er·a·tion
de·cen·tered
de·cid·ua
de·cid·u·ous
deci·gram
deci·li·ter
deci·me·ter
de·clive
de·col·or·ant
de·com·pres·sion
de·con·ges·tive
de·con·tam·i·na-
  tion
de·cu·ba·tion
de·cu·bi·tus
de·cus·sa·tion
de·den·ti·tion
def·e·ca·tion
def·er·ent
def·er·en·tial
de·fer·ves·cence
de·fi·cien·cy
def·i·ni·tion
de·for·mi·ty
de·gen·er·a·cy
de·gen·er·ate
de·gen·er·a·tion
de·glu·ti·tion
de·his·cence

de·hy·drate
de·hy·dra·tion
de·hy·dro·ge·nase
de·jec·tion
de·lim·i·ta·tion
de·lin·quen·cy
de·lir·i·um tre-
  mens
de·liv·ery
del·ta
del·toid *or* del·toi-
  de·us
de·lu·sion
de·mar·ca·tion
de·ment·ed
de·men·tia prae-
  cox
de·mul·cent
de·na·tur·ant
de·na·tured
de·ner·va·ted
de·ner·va·tion
de·ni·al
dens
den·si·ty
den·tag·ra
den·tal
den·ti·cle
den·ti·frice
den·tin *or* den·tine
den·tist·ry
den·ti·tion
den·toid
de·odor·ant
dep·i·late
de·pil·a·to·ry

dep·i·lous
de·pos·it
de·pres·sant
de·pres·sion
de·pres·sor
de·range·ment
de·riv·a·tive
der·ma
der·man·a·plas·ty
der·ma·ti·tis
der·ma·tol·o·gist
der·ma·tol·o·gy
der·ma·to·sis
de·scend·ens
de·scen·sus
de·sen·si·ti·za·tion
des·mi·tis
des·moid
des·qua·ma·tion
de·tach·ment
de·ter·gent
de·ter·mi·nant
de·ter·mi·na·tion
de·tri·tion
de·tru·sor
de·vi·a·tion
de·vi·tal·ize
dex·ter
dex·tral·i·ty
dex·trase
dex·troc·u·lar
dex·trose
di·a·be·tes
di·a·bet·ic
di·ag·nos·able *or*
  di·ag·nose·able

di·ag·no·ses pl.
di·ag·no·sis sing.
di·ag·nos·tic
di·ag·nos·ti·cian
di·am·e·ter
di·a·pho·re·sis
di·a·phragm
di·ap·la·sis
di·ar·rhea *or* di-
  ar·rhoea
di·as·ta·sis
di·a·stat·ic
di·a·ste·ma
di·as·to·le
di·a·stol·ic
dia·ther·my
di·ath·e·sis
di·chot·o·my
di·cum·arol
di·et
di·etary
di·etet·ics
dif·fer·en·tial
dif·frac·tion
dif·fuse
dif·fus·ible
dif·fu·sion
di·ges·tant
di·ges·tion
dig·it
dig·i·tal·is
dig·i·tal·i·za·tion
dig·i·tus
di·hy·brid
di·hy·drate
di·la·ta·tion

di·la·tion
di·la·tor
dil·u·ent
di·lute
di·lu·tion
di·men·sion
dim·ple
di·op·ter
di·op·tom·e·ter
di·or·tho·sis
di·ox·ide
diph·the·ria
dip·lo·coc·cus
dip·lo·pia
dis·charge
dis·col·or·ation
dis·crim·i·na·tion
dis·ease
dis·in·fec·tant
dis·in·fec·tion
dis·in·te·grate
dis·in·te·gra·tion
disk *or* disc
dis·lo·ca·tion
dis·mem·ber
dis·or·der
dis·pa·rate
dis·par·i·ty
dis·pen·sa·ry
dis·per·sion
dis·place·ment
dis·po·si·tion
dis·rup·tive
dis·sect
dis·sec·tion
dis·sec·tor

dis·sem·i·na·tion
dis·sim·u·la·tion
dis·so·ci·a·tion
dis·so·lu·tion
dis·solve
dis·sol·vent
dis·tal
dis·tance
dis·tem·per
dis·ten·sion *or*
　　dis·ten·tion
dis·til·late
dis·til·la·tion
dis·to·lin·gual
dis·to—oc·clu·sal
dis·tor·tion
di·ure·sis
di·uret·ic
di·va·ga·tion
di·ver·gence
di·ver·tic·u·lar
di·ver·tic·u·li·tis
di·ver·tic·u·lo·sis
di·ver·tic·u·lum
di·vi·sion
diz·zi·ness
doc·tor
dom·i·nance
dom·i·nant
do·nee
do·nor
dor·mant
dor·sal
dor·sum
dos·age
douche

dow·el
drachm
dra·gée
drain·age
Dram·a·mine
drib·ble
drop·per
drop·sy
drug·gist
drunk·en·ness
duct·less
duct·ule
duc·tus
du·ip·a·ra
dull·ness *or* dul·
　　ness
du·o·de·num
du·plic·i·ty
du·ra　ma·ter
dwarf·ism
dy·ad
dy·nam·ic
dy·na·therm
dys·acou·sia
dys·ar·thria
dys·ba·sia
dys·chi·ria
dys·chro·ma·top·
　　sia
dys·chro·mia
dys·cra·sia
dys·en·tery
dys·func·tion
dys·ki·ne·sia
dys·lex·ia
dys·lo·gia

21

dys·men·or·rhea
dys·met·ria
dys·mne·sia
dys·os·to·sis
dys·pep·sia
dys·pep·tic
dys·pha·gia
dys·pha·sia
dys·phe·mia
dys·pho·ria
dys·pla·sia
dys·pnea
dys·prax·ia
dys·sta·sia
dys·tax·ia
dys·the·sia
dys·thet·ic
dys·to·pia
dys·tro·phia
dys·tro·phy
dys·uria

E

ear·ache
eb·ur·na·tion
ec·cen·tric
ec·chon·dro·ma
ec·cy·e·sis
ec·dem·ic

ec·der·on
echid·nin
ech·o·la·lus
eclamp·sia
ec·ly·sis
ec·mne·sia
ecol·o·gy
eco·ma·nia
ec·sta·sy
ec·tal
ec·ta·sia
ec·thy·ma
ec·to·derm
ec·tog·e·nous
ec·to·pia
ec·to·plasm
ec·trom·e·lus
ec·tro·pi·on
ec·trot·ic
ec·ty·lot·ic
ec·ze·ma
ec·zem·a·to·sis
ede·ma
eden·tate
eden·tia
eden·tu·lous
ed·i·ble
ef·fec·tor
ef·fer·ent (away from
    center; cf. *afferent*)
ef·fer·ves·cence
ef·flu·ent
ef·flu·vi·um
ef·fu·sion
eger·sis
ego·cen·tric

ego·ma·nia
ejac·u·la·tion
ejec·tion
ejec·tor
elab·o·ra·tion
elas·tic
elas·ti·ca
el·bow
elec·tric·i·ty
elec·tro·car·dio·
    gram
elec·tro·car·di·
    og·ra·phy
elec·tro·cau·tery
elec·tro·cys·to·
    scope
elec·trode
elec·tro·en·ceph·
    a·lo·graph
elec·trol·y·sis
elec·tron
elec·tro·sec·tion
elec·tro·shock
elec·tro·ther·a·py
elec·tu·ary
el·e·ment
el·e·phan·ti·a·sis
elim·i·na·tion
elix·ir
elon·ga·tion
ema·ci·a·tion
emac·u·la·tion
em·a·na·tion
eman·ci·pa·tion
em·a·no·ther·a·py
emas·cu·la·tion

em·balm·ing
em·bed
em·bo·li pl.
em·bol·ic
em·bo·lism (condition caused by clot; cf. *embolus, thrombus*)
em·bo·lus sing. (moving clot; cf. *embolism, thrombus*)
em·bra·sure
em·bro·ca·tion
em·bryo
em·bry·ol·o·gy
em·bry·ul·cia
em·e·sis
emet·ic
em·e·tine
emic·tion
em·i·gra·tion
em·i·nence
em·is·sary
emis·sion
em·men·a·gogue
em·men·ia
em·me·tro·pia
emol·lient
emo·tion
em·pa·thy
em·phrax·is
em·phy·se·ma
em·phy·se·ma·tous
em·pir·ic
em·pir·i·cism
em·py·ema
em·py·e·sis

emul·si·fi·er
emul·si·fy
emunc·to·ry
enam·el
en·cap·suled
en·ceph·a·li·tis
en·ceph·a·lo·ma
en·ceph·a·lon
en·ceph·a·lop·a·thy
en·ceph·a·lor·rha·gia
en·cop·re·sis
en·cyst·ment
end·ar·te·ri·tis
en·dem·ic
en·der·mic
en·der·mo·sis
en·do·car·di·tis
en·do·car·di·um
en·do·cer·vi·ci·tis
en·do·cer·vix
en·do·cra·ni·um
en·do·crine
en·do·cri·nol·o·gy
en·do·cri·nop·a·thy
en·dog·e·nous
en·dog·e·ny
en·do·lymph
en·do·men·inx
en·do·me·tri·o·sis
en·do·me·tri·tis
en·do·me·tri·um
en·do·my·si·um
en·do·na·sal
en·do·neu·ri·um
en·do·phle·bi·tis

en·do·plasm
en·do·scope
end·os·te·um
en·do·the·li·o·ma
en·do·the·li·um
en·e·ma
en·er·gy
en·er·va·tion (failure of nerve energy; cf. *innervation*)
en·gorge·ment
en·large·ment
en·ta·sia
en·ta·sis
en·ter·al
en·ter·al·gia
en·ter·ec·ta·sis
en·ter·ec·to·my
en·ter·i·tis
en·ter·o·cele
en·tero·coc·cus
en·tero·coele *or* en·tero·coel
en·tero·co·li·tis
en·ter·o·cyst
en·ter·og·e·nous
en·ter·o·lith
en·ter·ol·y·sis
en·ter·on
en·ter·o·pexy
en·ter·op·to·sis
en·ter·or·rha·phy
en·ter·os·to·my
en·ter·ot·o·my
en·to·cele
en·to·cine

23

en·to·derm
ent·op·tic
ent·op·tos·co·py
ent·otic
en·tro·pi·on
en·tro·py
enu·cle·ate
en·ure·sis
en·vi·ron·ment
en·zyme
eo·sin·o·phil *or*
  eo·sin·o·phile
eo·sin·o·phil·ia
ep·en·dy·ma
ephe·lis
ephem·er·al
eph·i·dro·sis
epi·car·di·um
ep·i·cys·ti·tis
ep·i·dem·ic
epi·der·mis
ep·i·der·mi·tis
epi·did·y·mis
epi·gas·tric
epi·gas·tri·um
epi·glot·tis
ep·i·lep·sy
epi·my·si·um
epi·neph·rine
epiph·y·sis
epip·lo·on
ep·i·spas·tic
ep·i·the·li·o·ma
ep·i·the·li·um
ep·i·them
ep·u·lo·fi·bro·ma

equa·tion
equa·tor
equil·i·bra·tion
equi·lib·ri·um
equiv·a·lent
era·sion
erec·tor
er·ga·sia
er·gas·the·nia
er·gos·ter·ol
er·got
ero·sion
erot·ic
erot·i·cism
eruc·ta·tion
erup·tion
er·y·sip·e·las
er·y·the·ma
er·y·the·moid
er·y·thre·mia
eryth·ro·blast
eryth·ro·cyte
eryth·ro·der·ma
eryth·ro·phil
eryth·ro·sin
es·char
esoph·a·gos·to·my
esoph·a·gus
esoph·a·gram
es·sence
es·sen·tial
es·ter
es·ter·ase
es·the·sia
es·the·si·ol·o·gy
es·thet·ic

es·tra·di·ol
es·tri·ol
es·tro·gen
ether
ether·iza·tion
eth·ics
eth·moid
eth·nic
ethyl
eti·ol·o·gy
eu·ki·ne·sia
eu·pho·nia
eu·prax·ia
evac·u·a·tion
ev·a·nes·cent
ever·sion
evis·cer·a·tion
ex·ac·er·ba·tion
ex·al·ta·tion
ex·am·i·na·tion
ex·an·them
ex·ca·va·tion
ex·ca·va·tor
ex·ce·men·to·sis
ex·cip·i·ent
ex·cise
ex·ci·sion
ex·cit·abil·i·ty
ex·ci·tant
ex·ci·ta·tion
ex·clu·sion
ex·coch·le·a·tion
ex·co·ri·a·tion
ex·cre·ment
ex·cres·cence
ex·cre·ta

ex·cre·tion
ex·cur·sion
ex·cur·va·ture
ex·er·cise
ex·fo·li·a·tion
ex·ha·la·tion
ex·haus·tion
ex·hi·bi·tion
ex·hil·a·rant
ex·hu·ma·tion
ex·i·tus
exo·crine
ex·odon·tia
ex·odon·tist
ex·oph·thal·mos
ex·os·to·sis
ex·o·tro·pia
ex·pec·to·rant
ex·pec·to·ra·tion
ex·per·i·ment
ex·pi·ra·tion
ex·plan·ta·tion
ex·plo·ra·tion
ex·plor·a·to·ry
ex·pres·sion
ex·pres·siv·i·ty
ex·pul·sion
ex·san·gui·nate
ex·suf·fla·tion
ex·ten·sion
ex·ten·sor
ex·ter·nal
ex·tinc·tion
ex·trac·tion
ex·trac·tor
ex·tra·sen·so·ry

ex·tra·sys·to·le
ex·trav·a·sa·tion
ex·trem·i·ty
ex·trin·sic
ex·tro·phy
ex·tro·vert
ex·tru·sion
ex·u·date
ex·u·da·tion
eye·lid
eye·strain

F

fac·et
fa·cial (pertaining to face; cf. *fascial*)
fa·cies
fac·ul·ta·tive
faex
fal·lo·pi·an
fa·mes
fa·mil·ial
fa·nat·i·cism
far·a·dism
far·i·na·ceous
fas·cia
fas·cial (pertaining to tissue; cf. *facial*)
fas·cic·u·lus
fas·ci·ec·to·my

fas·ci·num
fas·ci·tis
fat·i·ga·bil·i·ty
fat·i·ga·ble
fa·tigue
fau·ces (aperture; cf. *foci, fossae*)
fau·na
fea·ture
feb·ri·fa·cient
feb·ri·fuge
fe·brile
fe·ces
fec·u·lent
fe·cund
fe·cun·da·tion
fe·cun·di·ty
fee·ble·mind·ed·ness
fe·male
fem·i·nism
fem·o·ral
fem·o·ro·tib·i·al
fe·mur
fe·nes·tra
fen·es·tra·tion
fer·ment
fer·men·ta·tion
fer·ric
fer·rous
fer·ru·gi·nous
fer·tile
fer·til·i·ty
fer·til·iza·tion
fes·ter
fe·ta·tion

fet·id
fe·tor
fe·tus
fe·ver
fi·ber *or* fi·bre
fi·bre·mia
fi·bril
fi·bril·la·tion
fi·brin
fi·bro·adenoma
fi·bro·an·gi·o·ma
fi·bro·blast
fi·bro·car·ci·no·ma
fi·bro·cel·lu·lar
fi·broid
fi·bro·ma
fi·bro·mus·cu·lar
fi·bro·myx·o·ma
fi·bro·pla·sia
fi·bro·sar·co·ma
fi·bro·sis
fi·bro·si·tis
fi·brous
fib·u·la
fil·a·ment
fil·ter
fil·trate
fil·tra·tion
fi·lum
fin·ger
fis·sion
fis·sip·a·rous
fis·su·la
fis·sure
fis·tu·la
fis·tu·li·za·tion

flac·cid
flat·u·lence
fla·tus
flav·i·cin
fla·vin
flex·i·ble
flex·ile
flex·or
flex·u·ous
flex·ure
floc·cu·la·tion
floc·cu·lent
floc·cu·lus
flor·id
fluc·tu·a·tion
flu·id·ounce
flu·o·res·cence
flu·o·ri·date
flu·o·ride
flu·o·ri·dize
flu·o·rin·a·tion
flu·o·rine
flu·o·ro·scope
flu·o·ros·co·py
fo·ci pl. (centers of
    morbid process; cf.
    fauces, fossae)
fo·cus sing.
fo·li·um
fol·li·cle
fol·lic·u·li·tis
fo·men·ta·tion
fon·ta·nel
fo·ra·men sing.
fo·ram·i·na *or*
    fo·ra·mens pl.

for·ceps
fore·arm
fore·fin·ger
fore·skin
form·al·de·hyde
for·mate
for·ma·tion
for·mu·la
for·ni·ca·tion
for·nix
fos·sa sing.
fos·sae pl. (depres-
    sions; cf. *fauces,
    foci*)
fos·sette
fos·su·la
found·ling
fo·vea
fo·ve·o·la
frac·tion·a·tion
frac·ture
frag·ile
fra·gil·i·ty
frag·men·ta·tion
frem·i·tus
fren·u·lum
fre·num
fren·zy
fre·quen·cy
fri·a·ble
fri·gid·i·ty
front·ad
fron·tal
fro·zen
fru·men·tum
frus·tra·tion

ful·gu·rat·ing
ful·gu·ra·tion
fu·lig·i·nous
ful·mi·nant
fu·mi·ga·tion
fun·da·ment
fun·dus
fun·gi (sing.: *fungus*)
fun·gi·cide
fun·gous adj.
fun·gus n. (pl.: *fungi*)
fu·ni·cle
fu·nic·u·lus
fu·nis
fur·ca
fur·cu·lum
fur·fur
fur·row
fu·run·cle (boil; cf. *carbuncle, caruncle*)
fu·run·cu·lo·sis
fus·cin
fu·sion

G

gait
ga·lac·tase
ga·lac·tin
ga·lac·toid

gal·e·o·phil·ia
gal·e·o·pho·bia
gall·blad·der
gall·stone
gal·van·ic
gal·va·ni·za·tion
gal·va·nom·e·ter
ga·mete
ga·meto·cyte
gam·ma
gan·glia pl.
gan·gli·on sing.
gan·gli·o·neu·ro·ma
gan·grene
gar·gle
gar·rot·ing
gas·tric
gas·tri·tis
gas·tro·cele
gas·tro·en·ter·ic
gas·tro·en·ter·ol·o·gist
gas·trol·o·gy
gas·tror·rha·gia
gas·trot·o·my
gauze
ga·vage n. (feeding by tube; cf. *lavage*)
ge·lat·i·fi·ca·tion
gel·a·tin
gel·so·ma
gem·i·na·tion
ge·na
gene
gen·era (sing.: *genus*)
gen·er·al

ge·ner·ic
gen·e·sis
ge·net·ic
ge·net·i·cist
ge·nial (mild)
ge·ni·al (of chin)
ge·nic·u·lar
ge·nic·u·late
gen·i·tal
gen·i·ta·lia
gen·i·to·uri·nary
ge·nome *or* ge·nom
ge·no·type
gen·tian
genu
gen·u·clast
ge·rat·ic
ger·a·tol·o·gy
ger·i·a·tri·cian
ger·i·at·rics
ger·mi·cide
ger·mi·na·tion
ger·o·der·ma *or* ger·o·der·mia
ge·ron·tic
ge·stalt
ges·ta·tion
gid·di·ness
gi·gan·tism
gin·gi·va sing.
gin·gi·vae pl.
gin·gi·val·gia
gin·gi·vi·tis
gir·dle
gla·brous
glan·des pl.

glans sing.
glau·co·ma
gle·noid
gli·o·ma
gli·o·sis
glob·ule
glob·u·lin
glo·bus
glom·era (sing.: *glo-mus*)
glo·mer·u·lo·ne-phri·tis
glo·mus (pl.: *glomera*)
glos·sa
glos·si·tis
glos·so·cele
glos·sop·a·thy
glos·sos·co·py
glot·tis
glu·cose
glu·ten
glu·te·us
glu·tin
glu·ti·nous
glut·tony
gly·ce·mia
glyc·er·in *or* glyc-er·ine
glyc·er·ite
glyc·er·yl
gly·cine
gly·co·gen
gly·co·ge·nase
gly·co·gen·e·sis
gly·col·y·sis
gly·co·nin

gly·co·pro·tein
gly·cos·uria
gly·cu·re·sis
gnat
gna·thal
gnath·ic
gnath·i·tis
goi·ter
goi·tro·gen·ic
gom·phi·a·sis
go·nad
go·nad·o·tro·phin *or* go·nad·o·tro-pin
go·nag·ra
go·nal·gia
gon·e·cyst
gon·e·pol·e·sis
go·ni·tis
go·ni·um
gono·coc·ci pl.
gono·coc·cus sing.
gono·cyte
gon·o·duct
gon·or·rhea
gon·y·on·cus
gouge
gout
gra·di·ent
grad·u·ate
gram—neg·a·tive
gram—pos·i·tive
grand mal
gran·u·la·tion
gran·ule
gran·u·li·form

gran·u·lo·cyte
gran·u·lo·ma
grat·tage
grav·id
grav·i·da
grav·i·ty
greg·a·rine
grume
gru·mous
gry·po·sis
guai·ac
guai·a·col
gu·ber·nac·u·lum
gul·let
gum·ma
gur·ney
gus·ta·tion
gus·ta·to·ry
gut·ta
gyn·an·dro·mor·phy
gy·ne·cic
gy·ne·col·o·gist
gy·ne·col·o·gy
gy·ne·co·mas·tia
gyn·i·at·rics
gy·rus

hab·it
ha·bit·u·a·tion

28

hal·i·to·sis
hal·lu·ces (sing.: *hal-lux*)
hal·lu·ci·na·tion
hal·lux (pl.: *halluces*)
halo·gen
ham·mer·toe
hang·nail
hap·lo·dont
ha·plo·pia
hap·lo·scope
hap·tics
hare·lip
har·mo·zone
haunch
head·ache
heal·ing
hear·ing
heart·burn
heart fail·ure
he·bet·ic
heb·e·tude
heb·e·tu·di·nous
he·ge·mo·ny
hel·coid
he·lic·i·form
hel·i·cis
he·li·um
he·lix
he·lo·ma
he·lot·o·my
he·ma·chrome
he·mal
he·man·gi·oma
he·mat·ic
he·ma·tin

he·ma·to·blast
hem·a·to·cele
he·ma·to·crit
hem·a·to·cyst
he·ma·tol·o·gist
he·ma·tol·o·gy
hem·a·to·ma
hem·a·tor·rhea
hem·a·tose
he·ma·to·sis
he·ma·to·zo·on
he·ma·tu·ria
hem·i·an·es·the·sia
hemi·a·nop·sia
hem·i·a·tax·ia
hem·i·bal·lism
he·mic
hem·i·cra·nia
he·min
hem·i·ne·phrec·to·my
hemi·ple·gia
hem·i·sec·tion
he·mo·blast
he·mo·cyte
he·mo·cy·to·blast
he·mo·dia
he·mo·glo·bin
he·mo·glo·bin·uria
he·mo·gram
he·mo·lith
he·mo·ly·sin
he·mol·y·sis
he·mo·my·e·lo·gram
he·mop·a·thy
he·mo·phil·ia

he·mo·phil·i·ac
he·mo·phil·ic
he·mo·pho·bia
he·mop·ty·sis
hem·or·rhage
hem·or·rhoids
he·mo·sta·sia
he·mo·stat·ic
he·mo·tho·rax
he·mot·ro·phe
he·par
hep·a·rin
hep·a·tec·to·my
he·pat·ic
hep·a·ti·tis
hep·a·ti·za·tion
hep·a·to·ma
hep·a·to·sis
her·biv·o·rous
he·red·i·ty
her·i·tage
her·met·ic
her·nia
her·ni·or·rha·phy
her·o·in (drug)
her·pes
het·er·o·cel·lu·lar
het·er·odont
het·er·og·e·nous
het·ero·graft
het·er·ol·o·gy
het·ero·mor·phic
het·ero·mor·phous
het·er·op·a·thy
het·er·o·phe·my
het·ero·phile

het·er·o·pho·ria
het·er·op·sia
het·er·o·scope
hex·a·chro·mic
hex·o·bar·bi·tal
hi·ber·na·tion
hic·cup *or* hic-
cough
hid·rad·e·ni·tis
hid·rad·e·no·ma
hid·ro·poi·e·sis
hid·ror·rhea
hi·dros·ad·e·ni·tis
hi·dro·sis
hi·drot·ic
hi·lar
hi·lus
hip·bone
hir·sute
hir·su·ti·es
his·ta·mine
his·ti·dine
his·tio·cyte
his·tol·o·gy
his·to·ma
his·tone
his·to·ry
his·to·tome
his·tot·o·my
hoarse
ho·do·pho·bia
ho·mi·cide
ho·mo·cen·tric
ho·mo·ge·neous
ho·mo·gen·ic
ho·mo·plas·ty

ho·mo·sex·u·al·i·ty
ho·ra
hor·de·o·la pl.
hor·de·o·lum sing.
hor·mone
hor·mo·zone
hos·pi·tal·iza·tion
hu·man
hu·mer·us
hu·mid·i·ty
hun·ger
hy·a·lin *or* hy·a-
line
hy·a·li·tis
hy·a·loid
hy·brid·iza·tion
hy·dra·gogue
hy·drate
hy·dra·tion
hy·drau·lics
hy·droa
hy·dro·cele
hy·dro·ceph·a·lus
hy·dro·chlo·ric
hy·dro·cor·ti·sone
hy·dro·gen
hy·drol·y·sis
hy·drom·e·ter
hy·drop·a·thy
hy·dro·pho·bia
hy·drops
hy·dro·ther·a·py
hy·dro·tho·rax
hy·dru·ria
hy·giene
hy·gien·ist

hy·gro·ma
hy·gro·scope
hy·gro·sto·mia
hy·men
hy·men·o·tome
hyo·glos·sal
hy·oid
hyp·al·ge·sia
hyp·ar·te·ri·al
hy·pas·the·nia
hyp·ax·i·al
hy·pen·gy·o·pho-
bia
hy·per·acid·i·ty
hy·per·ac·tiv·i·ty
hy·per·a·cu·i·ty
hy·per·al·ge·sia
hy·per·ce·nes·the-
sia
hy·per·chro·mat·ic
hy·per·chro·ma-
tism
hy·per·chro·ma·to-
sis
hy·per·di·crot·ic
hy·per·em·e·sis
hy·per·emia *or*
hy·per·ae·mia
hy·per·er·gia
hy·per·es·the·sia *or*
hy·per·aes·the·sia
hy·per·hi·dro·sis
hy·per·in·vo·lu·tion
hy·per·ker·a·to·sis
hy·per·ki·ne·sia
hy·per·me·tro·pia

30

hy·perm·ne·sia
hy·per·ne·phro·ma
hy·per·os·mia
hy·per·os·to·sis
hy·per·pi·e·sia
hy·per·pla·sia
hy·per·pnea
hy·per·py·rex·ia
hy·per·sen·si·tiv-
 i·ty
hy·per·som·nia
hy·per·ten·sion (high
 blood pressure; cf.
 hypotension)
hy·per·thy·roid-
 ism
hy·per·ton·ic
hy·per·tro·phy
hy·phe·mia
hyp·hi·dro·sis
hyp·na·gog·ic *or*
 hyp·no·gog·ic
hyp·nic
hyp·no·gen·ic
hyp·no·sis
hyp·no·ther·a·py
hyp·not·ic
hyp·no·tism
hyp·no·tize
hy·po·a·cid·i·ty
hy·po·ac·tiv·i·ty
hy·po·adre·nia
hy·po·cal·ci·fi-
 ca·tion
hy·po·cho·les·ter-
 e·mia

hy·po·chon·dri·ac
hy·po·chon·dri·a-
 sis
hy·po·chro·mic
hy·po·cone
hy·po·con·id
hy·po·cy·clo·sis
hy·po·cy·the·mia
hy·po·der·mic
hy·po·don·tia
hy·po·fer·re·mia
hy·po·func·tion
hy·po·gal·ac·tia
hy·po·glot·tis
hy·po·gly·ce·mia
hy·po·hi·dro·sis
hy·po·ki·ne·sia
hy·po·ma·nia
hy·po·mas·tia
hy·po·men·or·rhea
hy·po·me·tab·o-
 lism
hy·po·nych·i·um
hy·po·phos·phite
hy·poph·y·sis
hy·po·pi·e·sia
hy·po·prax·ia
hy·po·pro·sex·ia
hy·po·psy·cho·sis
hy·po·py·on
hy·po·sen·si·tiv·i·ty
hy·pos·mia
hy·po·som·nia
hy·po·spa·di·as
hy·po·sta·sis
hy·po·stat·ic

hy·pos·the·nia
hy·po·tax·ia
hy·po·ten·sion (low
 blood pressure; cf.
 hypertension)
hy·po·ten·sor
hy·po·thal·a·mus
hy·po·the·nar
hy·po·ther·mia
hy·poth·e·sis
hy·po·thy·mia
hy·po·thy·roid·ism
hy·pox·e·mia
hyp·ox·ia
hys·ter·ec·to·my
hys·ter·e·sis
hys·te·ria
hys·ter·o·cele
hys·ter·og·e·ny
hys·ter·oid
hys·ter·op·a·thy
hys·ter·o·scope
hys·ter·ot·o·my

I

ichor
ich·thy·oid
ich·thy·o·sis
ic·ter·ic
ic·ter·us

ide·ation
iden·ti·fi·ca·tion
ide·ol·o·gy
id·i·ol·o·gism
id·io·path·ic
id·i·op·a·thy
id·io·syn·cra·sy
il·e·itis
il·e·o·ce·cum
il·e·um (portion of
   small intestine; cf.
   ilium)
il·e·us
ili·a·cus
il·i·o·cos·ta·lis
il·i·o·fem·o·ral
il·i·o—in·gui·nal
il·i·um (upper part of
   hip bone; cf. *ileum*)
il·le·git·i·mate
ill·ness
il·lu·mi·na·tion
il·lu·sion
im·age
imag·i·na·tion
im·bal·ance
im·be·cile
im·be·cil·i·ty
im·bibe
im·bi·bi·tion
im·bri·ca·tion
im·ide
im·i·no
im·i·ta·tion
im·ma·ture
im·me·di·ate

im·med·i·ca·ble
im·mer·sion
im·mis·ci·ble
im·mo·bi·li·za·tion
im·mune
im·mu·ni·ty
im·mu·ni·za·tion
im·mu·no·gen·ic
im·mu·nol·o·gy
im·pac·tion
im·pal·pa·ble
im·ped·ance
im·per·a·tive
im·per·cep·tion
im·per·fo·rate
im·per·me·able
im·per·vi·ous
im·pe·ti·go
im·ping·er
im·plan·ta·tion
im·plants
im·po·tence
im·preg·nate
im·pres·sion
im·pro·cre·ant
im·pu·ber·al
im·pulse
im·put·abil·i·ty
in·a·cid·i·ty
in·ad·e·qua·cy
in·an·i·mate
in·ap·pe·tence
in·ar·tic·u·late
in—ar·ti·cu·lo—
   mor·tis
in·born

in·breed·ing
in·ca—bone
in·car·cer·a·tion
in·ca·ri·al
in·car·nant
in·cest
in·ci·dence
in·cin·er·a·tion
in·cip·i·ent
in·cised
in·ci·sion
in·ci·sor
in·ci·su·ra *or*
   in·ci·sure
in·cli·na·tion
in·co·ag·u·la·ble
in·co·her·ence
in·com·pat·i·ble
in·com·pe·tence
in·con·ti·nence
in·co·or·di·na·tion
in·cor·po·ra·tion
in·cre·ment
in·cre·tion
in·crus·ta·tion
in·cu·ba·tion
in·cu·ba·tor
in·cur·able
in·cus
in·da·ga·tion
in·de·cent
in·de·ci·sion
in·den·ta·tion
in·dex·es *or* in-
   di·ces
in·di·cant

in·di·ca·tion
in·di·ges·tion
in·di·go
in·di·rect
in·dole
in·do·lent
in·dol·og·e·nous
in·do·lu·ria
in·duc·tion
in·du·ra·tion
in·du·si·um
ine·bri·ant
ine·bri·a·tion
in·ebri·ety
in·ef·fi·ca·cy
in·er·tia
in ex·tre·mis
in·fant
in·fan·tile
in·farct
in·farc·tion
in·fec·tion
in·fe·cun·di·ty
in·fe·ri·or·i·ty
in·fer·til·i·ty
in·fes·ta·tion
in·fib·u·la·tion
in·fil·tra·tion
in·firm
in·fir·ma·ry
in·fir·mi·ty
in·flam·ma·tion
in·fla·tion
in·flec·tion
in·flu·en·za
in·fra·cla·vic·u·lar

in·frac·tion
in·fra·red
in·fric·tion
in·fun·dib·u·lum
in·fu·sion
in·ges·ta
in·ges·tion
in·gra·ves·cent
in·gre·di·ent
in·gui·nal
in·hal·ant
in·ha·la·tion
in·ha·la·tor
in·hal·er
in·her·ent
in·her·it·able
in·hi·bi·tion
in·hib·i·tor *or*
   in·hib·it·er
ini·tial
in·ject
in·jec·tion
in·ju·ry
in·lay·ing
in·nate
in·ner·va·tion (nerve
  supply of part; cf.
  enervation)
in·no·cent
in·noc·u·ous
in·nom·i·nate
in·oc·u·la·tion
in·op·er·a·ble
in·or·gan·ic
ino·si·tol
in·quest

in·sal·i·va·tion
in·sa·lu·bri·ous
in·san·i·tary
in·san·i·ta·tion
in·san·i·ty
in·scrip·tion
in·sec·ti·cide
in·se·cu·ri·ty
in·sem·i·na·tion
in·sen·si·ble
in·sert·able *or*
  in·sert·ible
in·ser·tion
in·sheathed
in·sid·i·ous
in·sight
in·sip·id
in si·tu
in·so·la·tion (sun-
  stroke)
in·sol·u·ble
in·som·nia
in·spec·tion
in·spi·ra·tion
in·spi·ra·tor
in·spi·ra·to·ry
in·spis·sant
in·sta·bil·i·ty
in·stance
in·step
in·stil·la·tion
in·stil·la·tor
in·stinct
in·stinc·tive
in·stru·ment
in·stru·men·ta·tion

33

in·suf·fi·cien·cy
in·suf·fla·tion
in·suf·fla·tor
in·su·lin
in·sus·cep·ti·bil·i·ty
in·te·gra·tion
in·teg·u·ment
in·tel·lect
in·tel·li·gence
in·tem·per·ance
in·tense
in·ten·si·fi·ca·tion
in·ten·si·ty
in·ten·tion
in·ter·car·pal
in·ter·cav·ern·ous
in·ter·cel·lu·lar
in·ter·cos·tal
in·ter·course
in·ter·den·tal
in·ter·dic·tion
in·ter·dig·i·ta·tion
in·ter·face
in·ter·fere
in·ter·fer·ence
in·ter·fol·lic·u·lar
in·te·ri·or
in·ter·lo·bar
in·ter·mar·riage
in·ter·max·il·lary
in·ter·ment
in·ter·mit·tent
in·ter·mus·cu·lar
in·tern
in·ter·nal
in·ter·nist

in·ter·os·se·ous
in·ter·os·se·us
in·ter·prox·i·mal
in·ter·space
in·ter·stic·es
in·ter·sti·tial
in·ter·trans·ver-
   sa·lis
in·ter·val
in·ter·vas·cu·lar
in·ter·ven·tric·u·lar
in·tes·ti·nal
in·tes·tine
in·ti·ma sing.
in·ti·mae or in·ti-
   mas pl.
in·toed
in·toe·ing
in·tol·er·ance
in·tox·i·cant
in·tox·i·ca·tion
in·tra—ab·dom·i·nal
in·tra·ar·tic·u·lar
in·tra·cel·lu·lar
in·tra·cys·tic
in·tra·group
in·tra·lo·bar
in·tra·lob·u·lar
in·tra·mus·cu·lar
in·tra·oral
in·tra·spi·nal
in·tra·uter·ine
in·tra·vas·cu·lar
in·tra·ve·nous
in·tra·ven·tric·u·lar
in·tra·ves·i·cal

in·trin·sic
in·tro·ces·sion
in·tro·flex·ion
in·tro·mis·sion
in·tro·spec·tion
in·tro·ver·sion
in·tro·vert
in·tu·ba·tion
in·tu·ba·tor
in·tus·sus·cep·tion
in·tus·sus·cip·i·ens
in·val·id adj.
in·va·lid n.
in·va·sion
in·ver·sion
in·vert
in·ver·te·bral
in·vet·er·ate
in·vi·ril·i·ty
in·vol·un·tary
in·vo·lu·tion
in·ward
io·dine
io·dism
io·dized
ion·iza·tion
ip·e·cac or ipe-
   ca·cu·a·nha
iras·ci·bil·i·ty
iri·dal
iri·dec·to·my
ir·i·de·mia
iri·des
ir·i·des·cence
ir·i·do·ki·ne·sia
iris

34

iri·tis
ir·ra·di·ate
ir·ra·di·a·tion
ir·ra·tio·nal
ir·re·duc·ible
ir·reg·u·lar·i·ty
ir·re·vers·ible
ir·ri·ga·tion
ir·ri·ga·tor
ir·ri·ta·bil·i·ty
ir·ri·ta·ble
ir·ri·tant
ir·ri·ta·tion
is·che·sis
is·chia pl.
is·chi·um sing.
isch·no·pho·nia
is·chu·ria
is·land
iso·cel·lu·lar
iso·chro·mat·ic
iso·chro·nal
iso·co·ria
iso·dont
iso·la·tion
iso·mer
isom·er·ide
isom·er·ism
iso·plas·tic
iso·tope
iso·trop·ic
is·sue
isth·mus
itch·ing
iter
ivo·ry

jac·ti·ta·tion
jac·u·lif·er·ous
jaun·dice
jaw·bone
jej·u·ni·tis
je·ju·ñum
joule
ju·gal
jug·u·lar
ju·men·tous
junc·tion
junc·tu·ra
jus·to ma·jor
ju·ve·nile
jux·ta·po·si·tion

kai·no·pho·bia
ka·olin
kao·pec·tate
ke·loid
ken·o·pho·bia

ker·a·tin
ke·ra·ti·nous
ker·a·ti·tis
ker·a·to·cele
ker·a·to·chro·ma·to·sis
ker·a·to·der·ma
ker·a·toid
ker·a·tol·y·sis
ker·a·tome
ker·a·tom·e·ter
ker·a·to·plas·ty
ker·a·to·scope
ker·a·tos·co·py
ker·a·to·sis
ker·a·tot·o·my
ke·rau·no·pho·bia
ke·to·sis
kid·ney
kilo·cal·o·rie
kilo·gram
kil·u·rane
ki·nase
ki·ne·mat·ics
ki·ne·si·at·rics
kin·es·the·sia *or*
kin·es·the·sis
ki·net·ic
ki·net·ics
ki·ne·tism
ki·ot·o·my
kleb·si·el·la
klep·to·ma·nia
knee·cap
knuck·le
ko·nim·e·ter

35

krau·ro·sis
kre·o·tox·ism
ky·pho·sis

L

la·bia (sing.: *labium*)
la·bile
la·bil·i·ty
la·bio·den·tal
la·bi·o·gin·gi·val
la·bi·um (pl.: *labia*)
la·bor
lab·o·ra·to·ry
la·brum
lab·y·rinth
lab·y·rin·thi·tis
lab·y·rin·thot·o·my
lac·er·at·ed
lac·er·a·tion (wound; cf. *maceration*)
la·cer·tus
lach·ry·mal *or* lac·ri·mal
la·cin·i·ate *or* la·cin·i·at·ed
lac·ta·tion
lac·te·al
lac·tic
lac·tif·er·ous

lac·ti·fuge
lac·tig·e·nous
lac·ti·su·gi·um
lac·tiv·o·rous
lac·to·ba·cil·lus
lac·to·gen
lac·to·gen·ic
lac·to·glob·u·lin
lac·tose
la·cu·na sing.
la·cu·nae *or* la·cu·nas pl.
lal·la·tion
la·lop·a·thy
lal·o·ple·gia
lamb·da
la·mel·la
la·mel·lar
lame·ness
lam·i·na
lam·i·nec·to·my
lan·ci·nat·ing
lan·guor
lan·o·lin
la·pac·tic
lap·a·rot·o·my
la·pis
lar·va sing.
lar·vae pl.
lar·vate *or* lar·vat·ed
la·ryn·geal
lar·yn·gis·mus
lar·yn·git·i·des pl.
lar·yn·gi·tis sing.
la·ryn·go·cele

lar·yn·gol·o·gy
lar·yn·gop·a·thy
la·ryn·go·scope
lar·yn·gos·co·py
lar·yn·got·o·my
lar·ynx (organ of voice; cf. *pharynx*)
las·civ·i·ous
lash
las·si·tude
la·ten·cy
la·tent
lat·er·al
lat·er·o—ab·dom·i·nal
lat·er·o·flex·ion
lat·er·o·pul·sion
lat·er·o·ver·sion
la·tis·si·mus
la·tus
la·vage (washing out of organ; cf. *gavage*)
la·va·tion
lav·en·der
lax·a·tive
lax·ity
lay·er
lay·ette
laz·a·ret·to *or* laz·a·ret
leach·ing
left—hand·ed
le·git·i·ma·cy
lei·o·der·ma·tous
lei·o·der·mia
lei·o·my·o·fi·bro·ma

lei·o·my·o·ma
lei·o·my·o·sar-
   co·ma
lei·ot·ri·chous
lei·po·me·ria
le·ma
lem·nis·cus
lem·on
le·mo·pa·ral·y·sis
le·mo·ste·no·sis
len·i·ceps
len·i·tive
lens
lens·om·e·ter
len·tic·u·lar
len·tic·u·late
len·ti·form
len·ti·glo·bus
len·ti·go
lep·er
lep·ro·ma
lep·ro·min
lep·ro·sy
lep·to·ce·pha·lia
lep·to·dac·ty·lous
lep·to·don·tous
lep·to·me·ninx
lep·ton
lep·to·spi·ra
lep·to·spi·ro·sis
lep·to·thrix
le·re·sis
les·bi·an·ism
le·sion
le·thal
le·thar·gic

leth·ar·gy
le·the
leu·cic
leu·cine
leu·ci·no·sis
leu·co·ma
leu·co·maine
leu·co·ma·i·ne·mia
leu·co·main·ic
leu·co·sin
leuk·ane·mia
leu·ke·mia
leu·ke·mic
leu·ke·mid
leu·ke·moid
leu·ko·blast
leu·ko·ci·din
leu·ko·cyte
leu·ko·cy·to·gen-
   e·sis
leu·ko·cy·to·poi-
   e·sis
leu·ko·cy·to·sis
leu·ko·cy·tot·ic
leu·ko·der·ma
leu·ko·ma
leu·kom·atous
leuk·onych·ia
leu·kop·a·thy
leu·ko·pe·nia
leu·ko·pe·nic
leu·ko·pla·kia
leu·kor·rha·gia
leu·kor·rhea
leu·ko·tome
leu·ko·trich·ia

leu·kot·rich·ous
leu·kous
le·va·tor
le·ver
lev·i·ta·tion
le·vo·duc·tion
le·vo·gy·rous
le·vo·pho·ria
lev·u·lose
lev·u·lo·se·mia
lib·er·a·tion
li·bi·do
li·bra
lice (sing.: louse)
li·cense or li-
   cence
li·cen·ti·ate
li·chen
li·chen·i·fi·ca·tion
lic·o·rice
lid·o·caine
lien
li·enal
li·e·nop·a·thy
li·en·tery
lig·a·ment
lig·a·men·tous
lig·a·men·tum
li·gate
li·ga·tion
lig·a·ture
lig·ne·ous
limb
lim·ber·neck
lim·bus
li·men

li·mes (pl.: *limites*)
lim·i·na
li·mi·nal
lim·i·tes (sing.: *limes*)
lim·i·troph·ic
li·moph·thi·sis
limp
lin·ea
lin·gua
lin·gual
lin·gu·la
lin·gu·lar
lin·guo·dis·tal
lin·guo·gin·gi·val
lin·i·ment
lin·seed
lin·tin
li·pa
lip·a·ro·trich·ia
lip·a·rous
lip·ec·to·my
li·pe·mia
lip·o·blast
lip·o·ca·ic
lip·o·cyte
lip·o·dys·tro·phy
lip·o·gen·e·sis
li·pog·e·nous
lip·o·gran·u·lo·ma
li·poid
lip·oi·dal
lip·oi·do·sis
li·pol·y·sis
li·po·ma
li·po·ma·to·sis
li·po·ma·tous

lip·o·me·tab·o·lism
lip·o·pe·nia
lip·o·phil
lip·o·phil·ia
lip·o·phre·nia
lip·o·sar·co·ma
lip·ping
li·pu·ria
liq·ue·fac·tion
liq·uid
li·quor
lisp
lis·te·ria
lis·ter·ine
li·the·mia
lith·ia
li·thi·a·sis
lith·ic
lith·i·um
lith·o·gen·e·sis
li·thog·e·nous
lith·oid
lith·o·labe
lith·o·ne·phri·tis
lith·o·phone
lith·o·scope
li·thot·o·my
lith·o·trite
lith·ous
lith·u·re·sis
lit·mus
lit·ter
liv·er
li·vid·i·ty
lo·bec·to·my
lo·bot·o·my

lob·ule
lob·u·li pl.
lob·u·lus sing.
lo·bus
lo·cal·iza·tion
lo·chia
lo·cho·per·i·to-
  ni·tis
lo·ci (sing.: *locus*)
lock·jaw
lo·co·mo·tion
lo·cum te·nens
lo·cus (pl.: *loci*)
log·ag·no·sia
log·am·ne·sia
log·a·pha·sia
log·o·ko·pho·sis
log·o·ma·nia
log·o·neu·ro·sis
log·op·a·thy
log·o·pe·dics
log·o·pha·sia
log·o·ple·gia
lon·gev·i·ty
lon·gi·lin·e·al
lon·gi·ma·nous
lon·gi·ped·ate
lon·gis·si·mus
lon·gi·tu·di·nal
lon·gi·typ·i·cal
lon·gus
loose·ness
loph·o·dont
lo·quac·i·ty
lor·do·sis
lo·tio

louse (pl.: *lice*)
lu·cid·i·ty
lu·cif·u·gal
lu·es
lu·e·tin
luke·warm
lum·ba·go
lum·bar
lum·bo·cos·tal
lum·bo·dor·sal
lum·bo·in·gui·nal
lum·bo·sa·cral
lum·bri·cal
lu·men
lu·mi·nance
lu·mi·nes·cence
lu·mi·nif·er·ous
lu·mi·nos·i·ty
lu·na·cy
lu·nate
lu·na·tic
lu·nu·la
lu·po·ma
lu·pus
lu·te·o·ma
lux·a·tion
lux·u·ri·ant
lux·us
ly·ing—in n.
lymph
lym·phad·e·nec·to·my
lymph·ad·e·ni·tis
ym·ph·ad·e·no·ma
ym·ph·ad·e·nop·a·thy

lym·pha·gogue
lymph·an·gi·o·ma
lym·phan·gi·tis
lym·phat·ic
lym·pho·blast
lym·pho·blas·to·ma
lym·pho·cyte
lym·pho·cy·to·ma
lym·pho·cy·to·sis
lym·pho·der·mia
lym·phog·e·nous
lym·phoid
lym·pho·ma
lym·pho·poi·e·sis
lym·phor·rhage
lym·phor·rhea
lyo·phile
lyo·pho·bic
ly·sim·e·ter
ly·sis
Ly·sol
ly·so·zyme
lys·so·dex·is

mac·er·a·tion (process of softening; cf. *laceration*)
mac·ra·cu·sia

mac·ro·cyte
mac·ro·cy·to·sis
mac·ro·lymph·o·cyte
mac·ro·mas·tia
mac·ro·me·lia
ma·crom·e·lus
mac·ro·scop·ic
mac·ros·mat·ic
mac·u·la
mad·a·ro·sis
mad·i·dans
ma·gen·bla·se
mag·en·stras·se
mag·ma
mag·ne·sia
mag·ne·sium
mag·ne·tism
mag·ni·fi·ca·tion
mag·num
maid·en·head
ma·ieu·si·o·pho·bia
ma·ieu·tics
maim
mal
ma·la·cia
mal·ad·just·ment
mal·a·dy
mal·aise *or* mal·ease
ma·lar
mal·as·sim·i·la·tion
ma·late
mal·di·ges·tion
mal·for·ma·tion
ma·lig·nant

39

ma·lin·ger·er
mal·in·ter·dig·i·ta·tion
mal·lea·ble
mal·le·o·li pl.
mal·le·o·lus sing.
mal·le·ot·omy
mal·le·us n.
mal·nu·tri·tion
mal·oc·clu·sion
mal·o·nate
mal·po·si·tion
mal·pos·ture
mal·prac·tice
mal·pres·en·ta·tion
mal·re·duc·tion
malt·ase
malt·ose
mal·turned
ma·lum
mal·union
mam·e·lon
mam·ma sing.
mam·mae pl.
mam·mal
mam·mal·gia
mam·ma·ry
mam·mec·to·my
mam·mi·form
mam·mil·la
mam·mil·la·ry
mam·mil·lat·ed
mam·mil·li·tis
mam·mose
mam·mot·o·my
ma·neu·ver

man·ga·nese
mange
ma·nia
man·ic
man·i·kin *or* man·ni·kin
ma·nip·u·la·tion
man·ni·tol
ma·nom·e·ter
ma·nu·bri·um
man·u·duc·tion
ma·nus
man·u·stu·pra·tion
ma·ran·tic
ma·ras·mus
marche—a—pet·it—pas
mar·gin·a·tion
mar·row
mar·ru·bi·um
mar·su·pi·al·iza·tion
mas·cu·line
mas·cu·lin·i·za·tion
mas·sage
mas·se·ter
mas·seur
mas·seuse
mas·so·ther·a·py
mast·ad·e·ni·tis
mast·ad·e·no·ma
mas·tal·gia
mas·tauxe
mas·tec·to·my
mas·tic
mas·ti·ca·tion

mas·ti·ti·des pl.
mas·ti·tis sing.
mas·toid
mas·toid·ec·to·my
mas·ton·cus
mas·top·a·thy
mas·to·sis
mas·tos·to·my
mas·tur·ba·tion
ma·ter·nal
ma·ter·ni·ty
mat·ing
ma·trix
mat·ter
mat·u·rate
mat·u·ra·tion
ma·ture
ma·tu·ri·ty
ma·tu·ti·nal
max·il·la
max·il·lo·fa·cial
max·il·lo·fron·ta·le
max·i·mal
max·i·mum
may·hem
maze
ma·zol·y·sis
mea·sles
mea·sure
me·a·ti·tis
me·atus
mech·a·nism
me·co·ni·um
me·dia
me·di·ad
me·di·al

40

me·di·an
me·di·as·ti·num
me·di·ate
med·i·ca·ble
med·i·cal
medi·care
med·i·cat·ed
med·i·ca·tion
med·i·ca·tor
me·dic·i·nal
med·i·cine
me·di·o·car·pal
me·di·o·dor·sal
me·di·o·fron·tal
me·di·o·tar·sal
me·di·um
me·di·us
me·dul·la
med·ul·lat·ed
med·ul·li·za·tion
meg·a·ce·cum
meg·a·coc·cus
meg·a·co·lon
meg·a·lo·blast
meg·a·lo·car·dia
meg·a·lo·cyte
meg·a·lo·ma·nia
mei·o·sis
me·la·gra
me·lal·gia
mel·an·cho·lia
mel·a·nin
mel·a·nism
mel·a·no·ma
mel·a·no·nych·ia
mel·a·no·phore

mel·a·no·sis
me·le·na or me·lae·na
me·li·tis
mel·i·tu·ria or mel·li·tu·ria
me·los·chi·sis
mem·bra pl.
mem·brane
mem·brum sing.
mem·o·ry
men·ac·me
men·ar·che
me·nin·geal
me·nin·ge·or·rha·phy
me·nin·ges (sing.: *meninx*)
me·nin·gi·o·ma
men·in·git·ic
men·in·gi·tis
me·nin·go·cele
me·nin·go·coc·cus
me·nin·go·cyte
me·nin·go·en·ceph·a·li·tis
me·nin·go·my·e·li·tis
me·nin·go·my·e·lo·cele
men·in·gop·a·thy
me·ninx (pl.: *meninges*)
men·is·cec·to·my
me·nis·ci (sing.: *meniscus*)

men·is·ci·tis
me·nis·co·cyte
me·nis·cus (pl.: *menisci*)
men·o·lip·sis
meno·pause
men·o·pha·nia
men·or·rha·gia
men·or·rhal·gia
men·or·rhea
men·o·sta·sia
men·o·stax·is
men·sa
men·ses
men·stru·ant
men·stru·a·tion
men·su·ral
men·su·ra·tion
men·ta (sing.: *mentum*)
men·tal
men·talis
men·ta·tion
men·thol
men·tum (pl.: *menta*)
me·phit·ic
me·ral·gia
me·ra·lo·pia
mer·cu·ma·til·in
mer·cu·ri·al
mer·cu·ric
Mer·cu·ro·chrome
mer·cu·rous
mer·cu·ry
mer·er·ga·sia
me·ris·tic

41

me·ro·pia
me·ros·mia
mes·a·or·ti·tis
mes·ar·te·ri·tis
mes·en·ceph·a·lon
mes·en·chyme
mes·en·ter·ec·to·my
mes·en·te·ri·um
mes·en·tery
me·si·o·buc·cal
mesio·clu·sion
me·si·o·dis·tal
me·si·o·gres·sion
me·si·o·in·ci·sal
me·si·o·la·bi·al
me·si·o·lin·gual
me·si·o—oc·clu·sal
mes·o·blas·te·ma
meso·car·di·um
meso·derm
mes·o·gas·ter
mes·o·ne·phro·ma
meso·neph·ros
mes·o·pexy
mes·o·phle·bi·tis
mes·o·rop·ter
meso·the·li·o·ma
meta·bi·o·sis
met·a·bol·ic
me·tab·o·lism
me·tab·o·lize
meta·car·pal
met·a·car·po·pha·lan·ge·al
meta·car·pus
meta·cone

meta·co·nid
meta·co·nule
met·a·dra·sis
met·al
me·tal·lic
meta·mor·phic
meta·mor·pho·sis
meta·mor·phous
meta·neph·ro·gen·ic
meta·pla·sia
meta·sta·ble
me·tas·ta·sis
me·tas·ta·size
meta·tar·sal·gia
meta·tar·sus
meta·troph·ic
me·te·or·ism
me·ter
meth·a·done *or*
    meth·a·don
meth·od
meth·yl
meth·y·sis
met·o·don·ti·a·sis
met·o·pan·tral·gia
me·top·ic
met·o·pon
met·o·pryl
met·ra·pec·tic
met·ra·to·nia
met·ra·tro·phia
me·trauxe
met·rec·ta·sia
me·tre·mia
me·tria
met·ric   sys·tem

me·tri·tis
me·tro·cele
me·tro·clyst
me·trop·a·thy
me·tro·phle·bi·tis
me·trop·to·sis
me·tror·rhea
me·tro·sal·pin·gi·tis
me·tro·stax·is
mi·celle
mi·cro·ab·scess
mi·crobe
mi·cro·bi·ol·o·gy
mi·cro·bi·ot·ic
mi·cro·bra·chia
mi·cro·cal·o·rie
mi·cro·chem·is·try
mi·cro·coc·cus
mi·cro·cyte
mi·cro·cy·to·sis
mi·cro·dont
mi·cro·gen·e·sis
mi·cro·li·thi·a·sis
mi·cro·ma·zia
mi·crom·e·ter
mi·cro·mil·li·me·ter
mi·cron
mi·cro·pho·nia
mi·crop·sia
mi·cro·pyk·nom·e·ter
mi·cro·pyle
mi·cro·scope
mi·cro·scop·ic
mi·cros·co·py

mi·cros·mat·ic
mi·cro·some
mi·cro·so·mia
mi·cro·steth·o-
 scope
mi·cro·sur·gery
mi·cro·tome
mi·crot·o·my
mi·cro·trau·ma
mi·cro·volt
mi·cro·wave
mic·tu·rate
mic·tu·ri·tion
mid·ax·il·la
mid·brain
mid·dle (halfway
 between; cf. *medial*)
mid·fron·tal
midg·et
mid·riff
mid·wife (pl.: *mid-
 wives*)
mi·graine
mi·grate
mi·gra·tion
mil·dew
mil·i·ar·ia
mil·i·ary
mi·lieu   ex·te-
 rieur
mi·lieu   in·te-
 rieur
mil·i·um
milk·ing
mil·li·am·me·ter
mil·li·am·pere

mil·li·cu·rie
mil·li·cu·rie—
 hour
mil·li·equiv·a·lent
mil·li·gram
mil·li·gram—hour
mil·li·li·ter
mil·li·me·ter
mil·li·mi·cron
mil·li·mol·ar
mil·li·mole
mil·li·nor·mal
mil·li·ruth·er·ford
mil·li·volt
mil·pho·sis
mi·me·sis
min·er·al
min·im
min·i·ma *or* min·i-
 mums pl.
min·i·mal
min·i·mum sing.
mi·nom·e·ter
mi·nor
mi·o·car·dia
mi·o·sis
mi·ot·ic *or* my·ot-
 ic
mir·ror
mis·an·thro·py
mis·car·riage
mis·car·ry
mis·ce
mis·ce·ge·na·tion
mis·ci·ble
mi·sog·a·my

mi·sog·y·ny
mi·sol·o·gy
miso·ne·ism
mite
mit·i·gate
mit·o·gen·e·sia
mi·to·sis
mi·tral
mix·ture
mne·mas·the·nia
mne·mon·ics
moan
mo·bil·i·ty
mo·bi·li·za·tion
mo·dal·i·ty
mod·el
mod·er·a·tor
mod·u·lus
mo·dus
mog·i·graph·ia
mog·i·la·lia
mog·i·pho·nia
mo·lar
mo·las·ses
mold·ing
mole
mo·lec·u·lar
mol·e·cule
mo·li·men
mol·li·ti·es
mol·lus·cum
molt
mo·ment
mo·men·tum
mo·nad
mon·ar·thric

mon·ar·thri·tis
mon·ar·tic·u·lar
mon·gol·ism *or*
   mon·go·lian·ism
mon·gol·oid
mon·i·li·a·sis
mon·i·tor·ing
mono·blast
mon·o·blep·sia
mon·o·coc·cus
mon·oc·u·lar
mo·no·cyte
mon·o·cy·te·mic
mono·cy·to·pe·nia
mono·cy·to·sis
mo·nog·a·my
mon·o·neph·rous
mon·o·neu·ri·tis
mo·no·nu·cle·o·sis
mo·no·pha·gia
mono·pho·bia
mono·phy·odont
mono·ple·gia
mon·o·tic
mon·ox·ide
mon·stros·i·ty
mon·tic·u·lus
mood
mor·bid
mor·bid·i·ty
mor·da·cious
mor·dant
morgue
mor·i·bund
mo·ron
mo·ron·i·ty

mor·phine
mor·phin·ism
mor·phol·o·gy
mor·sal
mor·sus
mor·tal·i·ty
mor·tu·ary
mos·qui·to
moth·er
mo·tile
mo·til·i·ty
mo·tion
mo·tor
mot·tling
mound·ing
move·ment
mu·cif·er·ous
mu·ci·lage
mu·cin
mu·cin·oid
mu·cip·a·rous
mu·co·cele
mu·co·cu·ta·ne·ous
mu·co—en·ter·i·tis
mu·coid (protein sub-
   stance; cf. *mucosa,*
   mucous, mucus)
mu·co·pu·ru·lent
mu·co·rif·er·ous
mu·co·sa (mucous
   membrane; cf. *mu-*
   coid, mucous, mucus)
mu·co·sal
mu·co·san·guin·e-
   ous
mu·co·se·rous

mu·co·si·tis
mu·co·stat·ic
mu·cous (pertaining to
   mucus; cf. *mucoid,*
   mucosa, mucus)
mu·cus (secretion of
   mucus membrane; cf.
   mucoid, mucosa, mu-
   cous)
mu·li·eb·ria
mu·li·eb·ri·ty
mul·ti·cel·lu·lar
mul·ti·grav·i·da
mul·ti—in·fec·tion
mul·ti·lob·u·lar
mul·ti·loc·u·lar
mul·tip·a·ra
mul·ti·par·i·ty
mul·ti·ple
mum·mi·fi·ca·tion
mum·mi·fied
mumps
mun·dif·i·cant
mur·mur
mus·cae vo·li·tan-
   tes
mus·cle
mus·cu·lar·i·ty
mus·cu·la·ture
mus·cu·lo·ten·di-
   nous
mus·si·ta·tion
mu·tant
mu·ta·tion
mute
mu·ti·la·tion

mu·tu·al·ism
my·al·gia
my·as·the·nia
my·a·to·nia (lack of
    muscle tone; cf.
    myotonia)
my·ce·to·ma
my·co·ci·din
my·coid
my·co·sis
my·de·sis
my·dri·a·sis
my·ec·to·my
my·e·lat·ro·phy
my·elin
my·e·li·nop·a·thy
my·eli·tis
my·e·lo·blast
my·e·lo·cyte
my·eloid
my·elo·ma
my·e·lo·ma·la·cia
my·e·lo·mere
my·el·on
my·e·lop·a·thy
my·e·lo·ple·gia
my·e·lo·scle·ro·sis
my·e·lo·sis
my·en·ta·sis
my·en·ter·ic
my·es·the·sia
my·lo·dus
my·o·blast
my·o·blas·to·ma
my·o·car·di·tis
myo·car·di·um

my·oc·lo·nus
my·o·cyte
my·o·dys·tro·phy
my·o·e·de·ma
my·o·ge·lo·sis
myo·glo·bin
my·o·glo·bi·nu·ria
my·o·ky·mia
my·ol·o·gy
my·o·ma
my·o·ma·la·cia
my·o·pal·mus
my·o·pa·ral·y·sis
my·o·pa·re·sis
my·o·path·ic
my·op·a·thy
my·ope
my·o·pia
my·o·por·tho·sis
my·or·rha·phy
my·o·sin
my·o·si·tis
my·o·su·ture
my·o·tac·tic
my·ot·a·sis
my·o·ten·o·si·tis
my·o·te·not·o·my
myo·tome
my·ot·o·my
myo·to·nia (excess of
    muscle tone; cf.
    myatonia)
my·ot·ro·phy
my·rin·ga
myr·in·gi·tis
myx·ad·e·ni·tis

myx·ede·ma
myx·ede·ma·tous
myx·id·i·o·cy
myx·o·cyte
myx·o·fi·bro·ma
myx·o·gli·o·ma
myx·o·ma
myx·o·ma·to·sis

na·cre·ous
nae·paine
nail
na·ked
nal·or·phine
na·nism
na·no·ceph·a·lous
na·noid
na·nom·e·lus
nan·oph·thal·mia
na·no·so·mia
na·no·so·mus
na·nus
nape
na·pex
na·phaz·o·line
naph·tha
naph·tha·lene

45

naph·thi·on·ic
naph·thol
naph·thyl
nar·ce·ine
nar·cis·sism
nar·co·anal·y·sis
nar·co·hyp·nia
nar·co·hyp·no·sis
nar·co·lep·sy
nar·co·ma
nar·co·ma·nia
nar·co·sis
nar·co·spasm
nar·cot·ic
nar·co·tine
nar·co·tism
nar·co·ti·za·tion
na·ris
na·sal
na·sa·lis
na·sal·ism
na·scence
na·scent
na·si·o·al·ve·o·lar
na·si·on
na·so·cil·i·ary
na·so·fron·tal
na·so·gen·i·tal
na·so·la·bi·al
na·so·la·bi·a·lis
na·so·lac·ri·mal
na·so·max·il·lary
na·so·pal·a·tine
na·so·phar·yn·gi·tis
na·so·pha·ryn·go-
 scope

na·so·pha·ryn·go-
 scop·ic
na·so·phar·ynx
na·so·scope
na·so·si·nus·i·tis
na·so·spi·na·le
na·so·tur·bi·nal
na·tal
na·tant
na·ti·form
na·tive
nat·re·mia
nat·u·ral
nau·sea
nau·se·ant
nau·se·at·ing
nau·seous·ness
na·vel
na·vic·u·lar
near·sight·ed·ness
ne·ar·thro·sis
neb·u·la sing.
neb·u·lar·in
neb·u·las or neb-
 u·lae pl.
neb·u·li·za·tion
neb·u·lize
neb·u·los·i·ty
ne·ca·tor
nec·a·to·ri·a·sis
nec·ro·bac·il·lary
nec·ro·bac·il·lo·sis
nec·ro·ba·cil·lus
nec·ro·bi·o·sis
nec·ro·cy·to·sis
nec·ro·cy·to·tox·in

nec·ro·gen·ic
ne·crog·e·nous
nec·ro·ma·nia
nec·ro·mi·me·sis
nec·ro·phil·ia
ne·croph·i·lism
nec·ro·pho·bia
nec·rop·sy
ne·crose
ne·cro·ses (sing.:
 necrosis)
nec·ro·sin
ne·cro·sis (pl.:
 necroses)
nee·dle
ne·en·ceph·a·lon
ne·frens
neg·a·tive
ne·glect
neg·li·gence
neis·se·ria
nem·a·to·da
Nem·bu·tal
neo·ars·phen·a-
 mine
ne·o—ar·thro·sis
ne·o·blast
ne·o·blas·tic
ne·o·cal·a·mine
neo·cer·e·bel·lum
ne·o·cin·cho·phen
neo·cor·tex
ne·o·cys·tos·to·my
neo·gen·e·sis
neo·ge·net·ic
ne·o·hom·bre·ol

ne·o·hy·drin
neo·my·cin
neo·na·tal
neo·nate
ne·oph·il·ism
neo·pho·bia
ne·o·phren·ia
ne·o·pine
neo·pla·sia
neo·plasm
neo·plas·tic
neo·stig·mine
neph·a·lism
neph·a·lis·tic
neph·e·lom·e·ter
neph·e·lo·met·ric
ne·phral·gia
ne·phrec·to·mize
ne·phrec·to·my
neph·ric
ne·phrit·ic
ne·phrit·i·des pl.
ne·phri·tis sing.
neph·ro·cap·sec·to·my
neph·ro·cap·su·lot·o·my
neph·ro·cyte
neph·ro·gen·ic
neph·ro·lith
neph·ro·li·thi·a·sis
neph·ro·li·thot·o·my
ne·phrol·o·gist
ne·phro·ma sing.
neph·ro·mas pl.
neph·ron

ne·phrop·a·thy
neph·ro·pexy
neph·ro·poi·e·tin
neph·rop·to·sis
ne·phror·rha·phy
neph·ro·scle·ro·sis
ne·phro·sis (disease of kidney; cf. *neurosis*)
ne·phrot·ic
ne·phrot·o·my
neph·ro·tro·pic
nerve
ner·vi (sing.: *nervus*)
ner·vine
ner·vos·i·ty
ner·vous·ness
ner·vus (pl.: *nervi*)
nes·ti·at·ria
nes·tis
neu·ral
neu·ral·gia
neur·apoph·y·sis
neu·ra·prax·ia
neur·as·the·nia
neu·rax·i·tis
neu·rec·ta·sia
neu·rec·ta·sis
neu·rec·to·my
neu·rec·to·pia
neur·en·ter·ic
neu·rer·gic
neur·ex·e·re·sis
neu·ri·a·sis
neu·ri·a·try
neu·ri·dine

neu·ri·lem·ma
neu·ri·lem·mi·tis
neu·ri·lem·mo·ma
or neu·ri·le·mo·ma
neu·ri·no·ma
neu·ri·tis
neu·ro·blast
neu·ro·blas·tic
neu·ro·blas·to·ma
or neu·ro·blas·to·ma·ta
neu·ro·ca·nal
neu·ro·chord
neu·ro·cir·cu·la·to·ry
neu·ro·coele *or* neu·ro·coel
neu·ro·cra·ni·um
neu·ro·crine
neu·ro·cu·ta·ne·ous
neu·ro·cyte
neu·ro·cy·to·ma *or* neu·ro·cy·to·ma·ta
neu·ro·de·al·gia
neu·ro·de·a·tro·phia
neu·ro·der·ma·ti·tis
neu·ro·der·ma·tro·phia
neu·ro·di·as·ta·sis
neu·ro·dy·nam·ic
neu·ro—e·lec·tro·ther·a·peu·tics
neu·ro·ep·i·the·li·o·ma

neu·ro·ep·i·the·li·um
neu·ro·fi·bril
neu·ro·fi·bro·ma
neu·ro·fi·bro·ma·to·sis
neu·ro·fi·bro·si·tis
neu·ro·gas·tric
neu·ro·gen
neu·ro·gen·e·sis
neu·ro·gen·ic
neu·ro·gen·i·cal·ly
neu·rog·e·nous
neu·ro·glan·du·lar
neu·ro·glia
neu·ro·gli·al
neu·rog·li·o·cyte
neu·rog·li·o·ma
neu·rog·li·o·ses pl.
neu·rog·li·o·sis sing.
neu·ro·gram
neu·ro·gram·mic
neu·rog·ro·phy
neu·ro·hu·mor·al
neu·ro·hyp·nol·o·gy
neu·ro·hy·poph·y·sis
neu·roid
neu·ro—in·duc·tion
neu·ro·log·ic
neu·ro·log·i·cal
neu·rol·o·gist
neu·rol·o·gize
neu·rol·o·gy
neu·ro·lymph
neu·rol·y·sin

neu·rol·y·sis
neu·ro·lyt·ic
neu·ro·ma
neu·ro·ma·to·sis
neu·rom·a·tous
neu·ro·mere
neu·rom·ery
neu·ro·mi·me·sis
neu·ro·mo·tor
neu·ro·mus·cu·lar
neu·ro·my·al
neu·ro·my·e·li·tis
neu·ro·my·on
neu·ro·my·o·path·ic
neu·ro·my·o·si·tis
neu·ron
neu·ro·nal
neu·ron·i·tis
neu·ro·nog·ra·phy
neu·ro·path·ic
neu·rop·a·thist
neu·ro·path·o·gene·sis
neu·ro·path·o·log·i·cal
neu·ro·pa·thol·o·gist
neu·ro·pa·thol·o·gy
neu·rop·a·thy
neu·ro·phys·i·ol·o·gy
neu·ro·pil
neu·ro·plasm
neu·ro·plas·mat·ic
neu·ro·plas·ty
neu·ro·pore

neu·ro·psy·chi·a·try
neu·ro·psy·chop·a·thy
neu·ro·psy·cho·sis
neu·ro·re·lapse
neu·ro·ret·i·ni·tis
neu·ror·rha·phy
neu·ror·rhex·is
neu·ror·rhyc·tes
neu·ro·sar·co·ma
neu·ro·scle·ro·sis
neu·ro·se·cre·tion
neu·ro·ses pl.
neu·ro·sis sing. (psy·chic disorder; cf. *nephrosis*)
neu·ro·skel·e·tal
neu·ro·spasm
neu·ro·spon·gi·um
neu·ros·po·ra
neu·ro·ste·ar·ic
neu·ro·sur·geon
neu·ro·sur·gery
neu·ro·su·ture
neu·ro·syph·i·lis
neu·ro·the·ci·tis
neu·ro·ther·a·py
neu·rot·ic
neu·rot·i·cal·ly
neu·rot·i·cism
neu·rot·me·sis
neu·roto·gen·ic
neu·ro·tol·o·gy
neu·ro·tome
neu·rot·o·my
neu·ro·tox·in

neu·ro·trau·ma
neu·ro·troph·ic
neu·ro·trop·ic
neu·ro·var·i·co·sis
neu·ro·vas·cu·lar
neu·ru·la *or* neu-
ru·lae
neu·tral·iza·tion
neu·tral·ize
neu·tral·iz·er
neu·tro·clu·sion
neu·tro·cyte
neu·tro·cyt·ic
neu·tron
neu·tro·pe·nia
neu·tro·phil *or*
neu·tro·phile
neu·tro·phil·ia
neu·tro·phil·ine
ne·vi (sing.: *nevus*)
ne·void
ne·vose
ne·vo·xan·tho—en-
do·the·li·o·ma
ne·vus (pl.: *nevi*)
new·born
nex·us sing.
nex·us·es *or* nex-
us pl.
ni·a·cin
nib·ble
nic·co·lum
niche
nick·el
nic·o·tine
nic·o·tin·ic

nic·ti·tate
nic·ti·ta·tion
ni·da·tion
ni·di *or* ni·dus·es
pl.
ni·dus sing.
night·mare
night sweat
ni·gres·cence
nig·ri·cans
ni·gri·ti·es
ni·gro·sine
ni·grous
ni·hil·ism
ni·o·bi·um
niph·a·blep·sia
niph·o·typh·lo·sis
nip·pers
nip·ple
ni·sus
nit
ni·ter
ni·trate
ni·tric
ni·trile
ni·trite
ni·tri·toid
ni·tri·tu·ria
ni·tro·gen
ni·tro·ge·nize
ni·trog·e·nous
ni·tro·glyc·er·in *or*
ni·tro·glyc·er·ine
ni·tro·mer·sol
ni·tro·syl
ni·trous

no·as·the·nia
No·car·dia
no·car·di·o·ses pl.
no·car·di·o·sis sing.
no·ci·cep·tive
no·ci·per·cep·tion
no·cive
noc·tal·bu·mi·nu·ria
noct·am·bu·la·tion
noct·am·bu·list
noc·ti·pho·bia
noc·tu·ria
noc·tur·nal
noc·u·ous
nod·al·ly
node
no·dose
no·dos·i·ty
nod·u·lar
nod·u·lat·ed
nod·ule
nod·u·li pl.
nod·u·lus sing.
no·e·mat·ic
no·ma
no·mad·ic
no·men·cla·ture
no·mo·gram
no·mo·graph
non·ac·cess
non·ad·her·ent
non·al·ler·gic
no·nane
non com·pos
men·tis
non·dis·junc·tion

non·elec·tro·lyte
no·ni·grav·i·da
non·in·fec·tious
no·nip·a·ra
non·lu·et·ic
non·ma·lig·nant
non·med·ul·lat·ed
non·mo·tile
non·mus·cu·lar
non·nu·cle·at·ed
non·oc·clu·sion
non·opaque
non·par·ous
non·pro·tein
non·re·straint
non·sex·u·al
non·spe·cif·ic
non·sup·pu·ra·tive
non·sur·gi·cal
non·vi·a·ble
no·o·psy·che
nor·adren·a·lin
nor·epi·neph·rine
nor·leu·cine
nor·ma sing.
nor·mae pl.
nor·mal·cy
nor·mal·i·ty
nor·mer·gy
nor·mo·blast
nor·mo·chro·mia
nor·mo·chro·mic
nor·mo·cyte
nor·mo·cyt·ic
nor·mo·cy·to·sis
nor·mo·gly·ce·mia

nor·mo·ten·sion
nor·mo·ten·sive
nor·mo·ther·mia
nor·mo·ton·ic
nor·mo·to·pia
nor·mo·vo·le·mia
nose·bleed
nose drops
nos·er·es·the·sia
no·sog·e·ny
no·sol·o·gy
nos·o·ma·nia
nos·o·pho·bia
No·sop·syl·lus
nos·o·taxy
nos·tol·o·gy
nos·top·a·thy
nos·to·pho·bia
nos·trate
nos·tril
nos·trum
no·tal
notched
no·ti·fi·ca·tion
no·to·chord
no·to·chord·al
no·vo·bi·o·cin
No·vo·cain
no·vo·caine
noxa sing.
nox·ae pl.
nox·ious·ness
nu·bile
nu·bil·i·ty
nu·cel·li pl.
nu·cel·lus sing.

nu·ces
nu·cha
nu·chal
nu·cin
nu·cle·ar
nu·cle·ase
nu·cle·ate
nu·cle·ation
nu·clei (sing.: *nucleus*)
nu·cle·ide
nu·cle·i·form
nu·cle·in
nu·cle·in·ase
nu·cle·of·u·gal
nu·cleo·his·tone
nu·cle·oid
nu·cle·o·li (sing.: *nu-cleolus*)
nu·cle·o·loid
nu·cle·o·lus (pl.: *nu-cleoli*)
nu·cle·on·ics
nu·cleo·plasm
nu·cleo·plas·mat·ic
nu·cleo·pro·tein
nu·cle·o·tide
nu·cle·us (pl.: *nuclei*)
nud·ism
nu·di·ty
nui·sance
nul·li·grav·i·da
nul·lip·a·ra sing.
nul·lip·a·ras pl.
numb
nu·mer·i·cal
num·mi·form

num·mu·lar
num·mu·la·tion
nun·na·tion
Nu·per·caine
nurse
nur·sery
nurs·ing
nurs·ling
nu·ta·tion
nu·ta·tory
nu·tri·ent
nu·tri·ment
nu·tri·tion·al·ly
nu·tri·tious
nu·tri·tive
nu·tri·to·ry
nu·tri·ture
nu·trix
nux
nyc·tal·gia
nyc·ta·lope
nyc·ta·lo·pia
nyc·ter·ine
nyc·to·phil·ia
nyc·to·pho·bia
nyc·to·pho·nia
nyc·to·typh·lo·sis
nyc·tu·ria
nymph
nym·pha sing.
nym·phae pl.
nym·phec·to·my
nym·phi·tis
nym·pho·lep·sy
nym·pho·ma·nia
nym·phot·o·my

nys·tag·mic
nys·tag·mi·form
nys·tag·mo·graph
nys·tag·mog·ra·phy
nys·tag·moid
nys·tag·mus

oa·sis
ob·ce·ca·tion
ob·dor·mi·tion
ob·duc·tion
obe·li·on
obese
obe·si·ty
ob·fus·ca·tion
ob·jec·tive
ob·li·gate
oblique
obliq·ui·ty
ob·li·quus
oblit·er·a·tion
ob·nu·bi·la·tion
ob·ses·sion
ob·ses·sive
ob·so·les·cence
ob·ste·tri·cian
ob·stet·ri·cal
ob·stet·rics
ob·struc·tion

ob·stru·ent
ob·tund·ent
ob·tu·ra·tion
ob·tu·ra·tor
ob·tuse
ob·tu·sin
ob·tu·sion
oc·cip·i·tal
oc·cip·i·ta·lis
oc·cip·i·to·ax·i·al
oc·cip·i·to·fron·tal
oc·cip·i·to·fron·ta·
lis
oc·cip·i·to·pos·te·
ri·or
oc·cip·ito·scap·u·
lar·is
oc·ci·put
oc·clu·sio
oc·clu·sion
oc·cult
oc·cu·pa·tion·al
oc·cu·pied
och·le·sis
och·lo·pho·bia
ochrom·e·ter
ochro·no·sis
oc·ta·caine
oc·tad
oc·ta·meth·yl·py·
ro·phos·phor·a·
mide
oc·tan
oc·tar·i·us
oc·ta·va·lent
oc·ti·grav·i·da

oc·tip·a·ra
oc·u·lar
oc·u·len·tum
oc·u·list
oc·u·lo·gy·ra·tion
oc·u·lo·gy·ric
oc·u·lo·mo·tor
oc·u·lo·my·co·sis
oc·u·lus
ocy·o·din·ic
odax·es·mus
odon·tal·gia
odon·tal·gic
odon·tec·to·my
odon·tex·e·sis
odon·tia
odon·ti·a·sis
odon·tic
odon·tin·oid
odon·ti·tis
odon·to·blast
odon·to·blas·to·ma
odon·to·cele
odon·to·chi·rur·gi·cal
odonto·cla·sis
odon·to·clast
odon·to·gen·e·sis
odon·tog·e·ny
odon·to·glyph
odon·to·gram
odon·to·graph
odon·tog·ra·phy
odon·to·hy·per·es·the·sia
odon·toid

odon·to·lith
odon·tol·o·gist
odon·tol·o·gy
odon·to·lox·ia
odon·tol·y·sis
odon·to·ma
odon·to·ne·cro·sis
odon·to·neu·ral·gia
odon·to·par·al·lax·is
odon·top·a·thy
odon·to·pri·sis
odon·top·to·sia
odon·tor·rha·gia
odon·tos·chi·sis
odon·to·schism
odon·to·scope
odon·tos·co·py
odon·to·sei·sis
odon·to·sis
odon·tot·o·my
odon·to·trip·sis
odon·tot·ry·py
odor·if·er·ous
odor·im·e·try
odyn·a·cou·sis
odyn·o·pho·bia
of·fal
of·fi·cial
of·fi·ci·nal
ohm·me·ter
oid·i·um
oi·ko·pho·bia
oi·no·ma·nia
oint·ment
olea
ole·cra·nar·thri·tis

ole·cra·nar·throc·a·ce
ole·cra·non
ole·o·mar·ga·rine
ole·om·e·ter
ole·o·ther·a·py
ole·o·vi·ta·min
ol·fac·tion
ol·fac·tom·e·ter
ol·fac·to·ry
ol·i·ge·mia
ol·i·ger·ga·sia
ol·ig·hid·ria
ol·ig·hy·dria
ol·i·go·blen·nia
ol·i·go·cho·lia
ol·i·go·chro·ma·sia
ol·i·go·chro·me·mia
ol·i·go·chy·lia
ol·i·go·cy·the·mia
ol·i·go·cy·the·mic
ol·i·go·dac·rya
ol·i·go·dac·tyl·ia
ol·i·go·den·dro·blas·to·ma
ol·i·go·den·drog·lia
ol·i·go·den·dro·gli·o·ma
ol·i·go·den·dro·gli·o·ma·to·sis
ol·i·go·don·tia
ol·i·go·dy·nam·ic
ol·i·go·el·e·ment
ol·i·go·ga·lac·tia
ol·i·go·gen·ic
ol·i·go·gen·ics

ol·i·go·hy·dram-
  ni·os
ol·i·go·hy·dru·ria
ol·i·go·me·lus
ol·i·go·men·or·rhea
ol·i·go·phos·pha-
  tu·ria
ol·i·go·phre·nia
ol·i·go·phren·ic
ol·i·gop·nea
ol·i·gop·ty·a·lism
ol·i·go·py·rene
ol·i·go·ria
ol·i·go·si·a·lia
ol·i·go·sper·mia
ol·i·go·trich·ia
ol·i·gu·ria
ol·i·vary
ol·i'·vif·u·gal
ol·i·vip·e·tal
ol·o·pho·nia
oma·gra
omar·thral·gia
omar·thri·tis
oma·sa pl.
oma·sum sing.
om·bro·pho·bia
omen·ta or omen-
  tums (sing.: omen-
  tum)
omen·tec·to·my
omen·to·pexy
omen·tor·rha·phy
omen·tum (pl.:
  omenta or omen-
  tums)

om·niv·o·rous
omo·cer·vi·ca·lis
omo·hy·oid
omo·ver·te·bral
om·pha·lec·to·my
om·pha·li (sing.:
  omphalos)
om·phal·ic
om·pha·li·tis
om·pha·lo·mes·en-
  ter·ic
om·pha·los (pl.:
  omphali)
om·phal·o·site
om·pha·lo·tax·is
om·phal·o·tome
om·pha·lot·o·my
om·pha·lo·trip·sy
onan·ism
on·cho·cer·ci·a·sis
on·cho·cer·co·ma
on·cho·der·ma·ti·tis
on·co·cyte
on·co·cy·to·ma
on·co·gen·e·sis
on·co·gen·ic
on·co·graph
on·cog·ra·phy
on·com·e·ter
on·com·et·ric
on·com·e·try
on·co·sis
on·co·sphere
on·cot·ic

onei·ric
onei·rism
onei·rol·o·gy
onei·ron·o·sus
onei·ros·co·py
onio·ma·nia
onio·ma·ni·ac
on·ion·peel
on·o·mato·ma·nia
on·o·mat·o·pho·bia
on·o·mat·o·poi·e·sis
ono·nis
on·to·ge·net·ic
on·tog·e·ny
on·y·chal·gia
on·y·cha·tro·phia
on·ych·aux·is
on·y·chec·to·my
on·y·chex·al·lax·is
onych·ia
on·y·chin
on·y·choc·la·sis
on·y·cho·cryp·to·sis
on·y·cho·dys·tro-
  phy
on·y·cho·gen·ic
on·y·cho·gry·po·sis
on·y·cho·hel·co·sis
on·y·cho·het·er·o-
  to·pia
on·y·choid
on·y·chol·y·sis
on·y·cho·ma
on·y·cho·ma·de·sis
  (loss of hair; cf. de-
  fluvium unguium)

on·y·cho·ma·la·cia
on·y·cho·my·co·sis
on·y·cho·pac·i·ty
(white spots within
the nail; cf. *leuk-
onychia*)
on·y·cho·path·ic
on·y·chop·a·thy
on·y·cho·pha·gia
on·y·choph·a·gist
on·y·cho·phy·ma
on·y·chop·to·sis
on·y·chor·rhex·is
on·y·chor·rhi·za
on·y·cho·schiz·ia
on·y·cho·stro·ma
on·y·chot·il·lo-
ma·nia
on·y·chot·o·my
onyx·i·tis
oo·cyst
oo·cyte
oo·gen·e·sis
oo·go·ni·um
oo·ki·ne·sis
oo·pho·rec·to·my
oo·pho·ri·tis
ooph·o·ro·cys·tec-
to·my
ooph·o·ro·cys·to·sis
ooph·o·ro·hys·ter-
ec·to·my
ooph·o·ron
ooph·o·ro·path·ia
ooph·o·ro·pexy
ooph·o·ro·plas·ty

ooph·o·ro·sal·pin-
gec·to·my
ooph·o·ro·sal·pin-
gi·tis
oo·pho·ros·to·my
oo·phor·rha·phy
oo·sperm
oo·tid
opaci·fi·ca·tion
opaci·fy
opal·es·cent
opa·les·cin
opaque
opei·do·scope
op·er·a·bil·i·ty
op·er·a·ble
op·er·a·tion
oper·cu·la pl.
oper·cu·lar
oper·cu·lum sing.
ophi·a·sis
ophid·i·o·pho·bia
ophid·ism
oph·i·o·phobe
oph·i·o·sis
oph·ry·i·tis
ophry·on
oph·ry·o·sis
oph·ryph·thei·ri-
a·sis
ophrys
oph·thal·ma·cro·sis
oph·thal·ma·gra
oph·thal·mal·gia
oph·thal·mec·chy-
mo·sis

oph·thal·mec·to·my
oph·thalm·en·ceph-
a·lon
oph·thal·mia
oph·thal·mi·a·ter
oph·thal·mi·at·rics
oph·thal·mit·ic
oph·thal·mi·tis
oph·thal·mo·cen-
te·sis
oph·thal·mo·co·pia
oph·thal·mo·di·ag-
no·sis
oph·thal·mo·di·a-
stim·e·ter
oph·thal·mo·do·ne-
sis
oph·thal·mo·dy·na-
mom·e·ter
oph·thal·mo·dyn·ia
oph·thal·mo·fun-
do·scope
oph·thal·mog·ra-
phy
oph·thal·mo·gy·ric
oph·thal·mo·i·co-
nom·e·ter
oph·thal·mo·leu-
ko·scope
oph·thal·mo·lith
oph·thal·mo·log·ic
oph·thal·mol·o·gist
oph·thal·mol·o·gy
oph·thal·mo·ly·ma
oph·thal·mo·ma-
cro·sis

oph·thal·mo·ma·la·cia

oph·thal·mo·mel·a·no·ma

oph·thal·mo·mel·a·no·sis

oph·thal·mom·e·ter

oph·thal·mom·e·try

oph·thal·mo·my·co·sis

oph·thal·mo·my·ia·sis

oph·thal·mo·my·i·tis

oph·thal·mo·neu·ri·tis

oph·thal·mop·a·thy

oph·thal·mo·pha·com·e·ter

oph·thal·mo·phas·ma·tos·co·py

oph·thal·mo·pho·bia

oph·thal·moph·thi·sis

oph·thal·mo·phy·ma

oph·thal·mo·plas·ty

oph·thal·mo·ple·gia

oph·thal·mo·ple·gic

oph·thal·mop·to·sis

oph·thal·mo—re·ac·tion

oph·thal·mor·rha·gia

oph·thal·mor·rhea

oph·thal·mor·rhex·is

oph·thal·mos

oph·thal·mo·scope

oph·thal·mo·scop·ic

oph·thal·mos·co·pist

oph·thal·mos·co·py

oph·thal·mo·spasm

oph·thal·mo·spin·ther·ism

oph·thal·mos·ta·sis

oph·thal·mo·stat

oph·thal·mo·sta·tom·e·ter

oph·thal·mo·sta·tom·e·try

oph·thal·mo·ste·re·sis

oph·thal·mo·syn·chy·sis

oph·thal·mo·ther·mom·e·ter

oph·thal·mot·o·my

oph·thal·mo·to·nom·e·ter

oph·thal·mo·to·nom·e·try

oph·thal·mo·trope

oph·thal·mo·tro·pom·e·ter

oph·thal·mo·tro·pom·e·try

oph·thal·mo·vas·cu·lar

oph·thal·mox·ys·ter

oph·thal·mox·ys·trum

oph·thal·mu·la

opi·ate

opi·o·ma·nia

opi·o·pha·gia

opio·phile

opis·then

opis·the·nar

opis·thia pl.

opis·thi·on sing.

opis·tho·cra·ni·on

op·is·thog·na·thism

opis·tho·po·reia

opis·thor·chi·a·sis

opis·tho·ton·ic

op·is·thot·o·nos

opi·um

op·o·del·doc

op·pi·la·tion

op·po·nens

op·sig·e·nes

op·sin·o·gen

op·si·nog·e·nous

op·si·o·no·sis

op·so·ma·nia

op·so·ma·niac

op·so·nin

op·so·nize

op·so·no·cy·to·pha·gic

op·son·o·ther·a·py

op·tes·the·sia

op·tic

op·ti·cal

55

op·ti·cian
op·ti·co·chi·as-
   mat·ic
op·ti·co·cil·i·ary
op·ti·coel
op·ti·co·pu·pil·lary
op·tics
op·tim·e·ter
op·ti·mum
op·to·gram
op·tom·e·ter
op·tom·e·trist
op·tom·e·try
op·to·my·om·e·ter
op·to·type
ora
orad
oral
ora·le
or·bic·u·lar
or·bic·u·la·re
or·bi·cu·lar·is
or·bi·tale
or·bi·ta·lia
or·bi·to·na·sal
or·bi·to·nom·e·ter
or·bi·to·sphe·noid
or·bi·tot·o·my
or·ce·in
or·chic
or·chi·dop·a·thy
or·chid·o·plas·ty
or·chi·dot·o·my
or·chi·ec·to·my
or·chi·en·ceph·a-
   lo·ma

or·chi·ep·i·did·y-
   mi·tis
or·chi·o·ca·tab·a·sis
or·chi·o·cele
or·chi·op·a·thy
or·chi·o·pexy
or·chi·o·plas·ty
or·chis
or·chit·ic
or·chi·tis
or·der·ly
or·di·nate
or·e·go·nen·sin
orex·is
or·gan·elle
or·gan·ic
or·gan·ism
or·ga·ni·za·tion
or·gan·o·gen·e·sis
or·gan·o·ge·net·ic
or·gan·oid
or·gan·ol·o·gy
or·ga·nos·co·py
or·gano·sol
or·gan·o·ther·a·py
or·gano·troph·ic
or·gan·o·trop·ic
or·gan·ot·ro·pism
or·gan·ot·ro·py
or·gasm
or·gas·mo·lep·sy
ori·en·ta·tion
or·i·fice
or·i·fi·cial
or·i·gin
or·ni·thine

or·ni·thod·o·rus
or·ni·thyl
oro·phar·ynx
or·o·sin
or·phol
or·pi·ment
or·rho·men·in·gi·tis
or·rhos
or·ris
or·thi·auch·e·nus
or·thi·o·chor·dus
or·thi·o·cor·y·phus
or·thi·o·don·tus
or·thi·o·me·to·pus
or·thi·o·pis·thi·us
or·thi·o·pis·tho-
   cra·ni·us
or·thi·o·pro·so·pus
or·thi·op·y·lus
or·thi·or·rhi·nus
or·thi·u·ra·nis·cus
or·tho·bo·ric
or·tho·caine
or·tho·ceph·a·ly
or·tho·chlo·ro-
   phe·nol
or·tho·cho·rea
or·tho·cre·sol
or·tho·dac·ty·lous
or·tho·den·tin
or·tho·di·a·gram
or·tho·di·a·graph
or·tho·di·ag·ra·phy
orth·odon·tics
orth·odon·tist
or·tho·gen·e·sis

or·tho·ge·net·ic
or·tho·gen·ic
or·thog·nath·ic
or·tho·grade
or·tho·mes·o·ceph-
a·lous
or·thom·e·ter
or·tho·pe·dic
or·tho·pe·dics
or·tho·pe·dist
or·tho·per·cus·sion
or·tho·pho·ria
or·thop·nea
or·thop·ne·ic
or·tho·prax·is
or·tho·psy·chi·a·try
or·thop·tera
or·thop·tic
or·thop·tics
or·thop·to·scope
or·tho·scope
or·tho·scop·ic
or·thos·co·py
or·tho·sis
or·tho·tast
or·tho·ter·i·on
or·tho·tic
or·tho·ton·ic
or·thot·o·nus
or·tho·trop·ic
or·thot·ro·pism
os (pl.: *ossa*)
osa·zone
os·chea
os·cheal
os·cil·la·tion

os·cil·la·tor
os·cil·lo·graph
os·cil·lom·e·ter
os·cil·lo·met·ric
os·cil·lom·e·try
os·cil·lop·sia
os·cil·lo·scope
os·ci·tan·cy
os·ci·ta·tion
os·cu·la pl.
os·cu·la·tion
os·cu·lum sing.
os·mat·ic
os·mes·the·sia
os·mic
os·mi·dro·sis
os·mi·um
os·mo·dys·pho·ria
os·mol
os·mo·lar·i·ty
os·mol·o·gy
os·mom·e·ter
os·mo·pho·bia
os·mo·phore
os·mo·re·cep·tor
os·mo·reg·u·lar·i·ty
os·mo·sis
os·mot·ic
os·phre·si·om·e·ter
os·sa (sing.: *os*)
os·se·in
os·se·o·al·bu·mi-
noid
os·se·o·car·ti·lag·i-
nous
os·se·o·fi·brous

os·se·o·mu·coid
os·se·ous
os·si·cle
os·si·cu·lec·to·my
os·si·cu·lot·o·my
os·sif·er·ous
os·sif·ic
os·si·fi·ca·tion
os·sif·lu·ent
os·si·form
os·si·fy
os·tal·gia
os·te·al
os·te·al·le·o·sis
os·te·an·a·gen·e·sis
os·te·a·naph·y·sis
os·tec·to·my
os·tec·to·py
os·te·it·ic
os·te·itis
os·tem·py·e·sis
os·teo·an·eu·rysm
os·teo·ar·thri·tis
os·teo·ar·throp·a-
thy
os·teo·ar·throt·o·my
os·teo·blast
os·teo·blas·tic
os·te·o·blas·to·ma
os·te·o·car·ci·no·ma
os·te·o·car·ti·lag·i-
nous
os·te·o·chon·dral
os·te·o·chon·dri·tis
os·te·o·chon·dro-
dys·pla·sia

57

os·te·o·chon·dro·ma
os·te·o·chon·dro·ma·to·sis
os·te·o·chon·dro·sar·co·ma
os·te·o·chon·dro·sis
os·te·oc·la·sis
os·te·o·clast
os·te·o·clas·to·ma
os·te·o·cys·to·ma
os·te·o·cyte
os·te·o·den·tin
os·te·o·der·ma·to·plas·tic
os·te·o·der·mia
os·te·o·dyn·ia
os·te·o·dys·tro·phy
os·te·o·fi·bro·li·po·ma
os·te·o·fi·bro·ma
os·te·o·gen
os·te·o·gen·e·sis
os·te·o·gen·ic
os·te·og·e·nous
os·te·o·hy·per·troph·ic
os·te·oid
os·te·o·lip·o·chon·dro·ma
os·te·o·lith
os·te·ol·o·gy
os·te·ol·y·sis
os·te·o·ma
os·te·o·ma·la·cia
os·te·o·met·ric
os·te·om·e·try

os·teo·my·e·lit·ic
os·teo·my·eli·tis
os·te·o·my·e·log·ra·phy
os·te·o·ne·cro·sis
os·te·o·neph·rop·a·thy
os·teo·path
os·te·o·path·ia
os·teo·path·ic
os·te·op·a·thy
os·te·o·phage
os·te·o·oph·o·ny
os·te·o·phyte
os·te·o·plaque
os·teo·plas·tic
os·teo·plas·ty
os·te·o·poi·ki·lo·sis
os·teo·po·ro·sis
os·te·o·ra·di·o·ne·cro·sis
os·teo·sar·co·ma
os·te·o·sar·co·ma·tous
os·te·o·sis
os·te·o·spon·gi·o·ma
os·te·o·stix·is
os·te·o·su·ture
os·te·o·syn·o·vi·tis
os·teo·syn·the·sis
os·te·o·ta·bes
os·te·o·throm·bo·sis
os·te·o·tome
os·te·o·to·mo·cla·sia

os·te·o·to·moc·la·sis
os·te·ot·o·my
os·te·o·tribe
os·te·ot·ro·phy
os·tia pl.
os·ti·al
os·ti·um sing.
otal·gia
otan·tri·tis
othe·ma·to·ma
ot·hem·or·rha·gia
ot·hem·or·rhea
otic
oti·co·din·ia
otit·i·des pl.
oti·tis sing.
oto·blen·or·rhea
oto·clei·sis
oto·cyst
oto·cys·tic
oto·dyn·ia
oto·gen·ic
otog·e·nous
oto·hem·i·neur·as·the·nia
oto·lar·yn·gol·o·gist
oto·lar·yn·gol·o·gy
oto·log·ic
oto·log·i·cal·ly
otol·o·gist
otol·o·gy
oto·my·as·the·nia
oto·my·co·sis
oto·my·cot·ic
oto·neur·as·the·nia

oto·pha·ryn·ge·al
oto·plas·ty
oto·pol·y·pus
oto·py·or·rhea
oto·py·o·sis
oto·rhi·nol·o·gy
otor·rha·gia
otor·rhea
oto·scle·ro·sis
oto·scle·ro·tic
oto·scope
oto·scop·ic
otos·co·py
otot·o·my
oto·tox·ic
otri·vin
ou·loid
ou·lor·rha·gia
ounce
out·let
out·limb
out·pa·tient
ova (sing.: *ovum*)
oval
ov·al·bu·min
ovalo·cyte
ovalo·cy·to·ses pl.
ovalo·cy·to·sis sing.
ovar·ia (sing.: *ovarium*)
ovari·al·gia
ovar·i·an
ovari·ec·to·my
ovari·o·cele
ovari·o·cen·te·sis

ovari·o·cy·e·sis
ovari·o·dys·neu·ria
ovari·o·gen·ic
ovari·o·hys·ter-
ec·to·my
ovari·o·lyt·ic
ovari·or·rhex·is
ovar·i·ot·o·my
ovari·o·tu·bal
ova·rit·i·des pl.
ova·ri·tis sing.
ovar·i·um (pl.: *ovaria*)
ova·ry
over·bite
over·cor·rec·tion
over·de·pen·den·cy
over·de·ter·mi·na-
tion
over·dose n., v.
over·flow
over·growth
over·jet
over·ly·ing
over·max·i·mal
over·rid·ing
over·strain
over·tone
over·weight
ovi·du·cal
ovi·duct
ovi·duc·tal
ovif·er·ous
ovi·fi·ca·tion
ovi·form
ovi·gen·e·sis

ovi·germ
ovig·er·ous
ovip·a·ra sing.
ovip·a·rae pl.
ovip·a·rous
ovi·pos·it
ovi·po·si·tion
ovi·vi·tel·lus
ovo·cen·ter
ovo·fla·vin
ovo·glob·u·lin
ovoid
ovoi·dal
ovo·mu·cin
ovo·mu·coid
ovo·plasm
ovo·plas·mic
ovo·tes·tis
ovo·vi·tel·lin
ovu·la (sing.: *ovulum*)
ovu·lar
ovu·la·tion
ovule
ovu·lif·er·ous
ovu·log·e·nous
ovu·lum (pl.: *ovula*)
ovum (pl.: *ova*)
ox·a·late
ox·a·le·mia
ox·al·ic
ox·al·ism
ox·al·o·sis
ox·al·uria
ox·a·zine
ox·i·dant
ox·i·dase

ox·i·da·tion
ox·ide
ox·i·dize
ox·ime
ox·im·e·ter
ox·i·met·ric
oxy·a·phia
oxy·blep·sia
oxy·ceph·a·ly
oxy·es·the·sia
ox·y·gen
ox·y·gen·ase
ox·y·gen·at·ed
ox·y·gen·ation
ox·y·geu·sia
ox·y·la·lia
ox·y·mel
oxy·mo·ron
ox·yn·tic
oxy·opia sing.
oxy·opias pl.
oxy·op·ter
oxy·os·phre·sia
oxy·phe·no·ni·um
oxy·phile or oxy-
    phil or
    oxy·phil·ic
    or ox·yph·i·lous
oxy·pho·nia
oxy·rhine
ox·y·to·cia
oxy·to·cic
oxy·to·cin
oxy·urid
oze·na or ozoe·na
ozo·chro·tia

ozoch·ro·tous
ozo·ke·rite or
    ozo·ce·rite
ozo·sto·mia

pab·lum
pab·u·lum
pace·mak·er
pachy·ac·ria
pachy·bleph·a·ron
pachy·bleph·a·ro·sis
pachy·ce·pha·lia or
    pachy·ce·pha·ly
pachy·ce·phal·ic
pachy·chei·lia
pachy·dac·ty·lia
pachy·der·ma·tous
pachy·der·mia
pachy·der·mi·al
pachy·e·mia
pachy·glos·sal or
    pachy·glos·sate
pachy·hem·a·tous
pachy·lep·to·men-
    in·gi·tis
pachy·lo·sis
pachy·me·nin·ges
pachy·men·in·git·ic

pachy·men·in·gi·tis
pachy·men·in·gop-
    a·thy
pachy·me·ninx
pa·chyn·sis
pachy·o·nych·ia
pachy·o·tia
pachy·per·i·to·ni·tis
pa·chyp·o·dous
pachy·tene
pa·chyt·ri·chous
pachy·vag·i·ni·tis
pac·i·fi·er
pac·ing
pa·go·plex·ia
pain
pal·a·ta (sing.: pala-
    tum)
pal·a·tal
pal·ate
pal·a·tine
pal·a·ti·tis
pal·a·to·glos·sal
pal·a·to·glos·sus
pal·a·to·max·il·lary
pal·a·to·na·sal
pal·a·to·pha·ryn-
    ge·us
pal·a·to·ple·gia
pal·a·to·prox·i·mal
pal·a·to·pter·y·goid
pal·a·tor·rha·phy
pal·a·to·sal·pin-
    ge·us
pal·a·tos·chi·sis
pal·a·tum (pl.: palata)

pa·le·en·ceph·a·lon
pa·leo·cer·e·bel·lum
pa·leo·pal·li·um
pal·i·ki·ne·sia
pali·la·lia
pal·in·dro·mia
pal·in·dro·mi·cal·ly
pal·inm·ne·sis
pal·i·phra·sia
pal·ir·rhea
pal·la·di·um
pall·an·es·the·sia
pall·es·the·sia
pal·lia pl.
pal·li·ate
pal·li·a·tion
pal·lia·tive
pal·lid
pal·li·dal
pal·li·um sing.
pal·lor
palm
pal·mar
pal·mar·is
pal·ma·ture
pal·mi·ped
pal·mi·tate
pal·mit·ic
pal·mod·ic
pal·mo·spas·mus
pal·mus
pal·pa·ble
pal·pate
pal·pa·tion (location by touch; cf. *palpitation*)

pal·pe·bra
pal·pe·bral
pal·pe·bra·lis
pal·pe·brate
pal·pe·bra·tion
pal·pi·tant
pal·pi·tate
pal·pi·ta·tion (rapid heart action; cf. *palpation*)
pal·sied
pal·sy
pan·a·cea
pan·ag·glu·ti·na·tion
pan·ag·glu·ti·nin
pan·ar·te·ri·tis
pan·ar·thri·tis
pan·at·ro·phy
pan·car·di·tis
pan·co·lec·to·my
pan·cre·as sing.
pan·cre·a·ta pl.
pan·cre·a·tec·to·my
pan·cre·at·ic
pan·cre·at·i·co·du·o·de·nal
pan·cre·at·i·co—en·ter·os·to·my
pan·cre·at·i·co·gas·tros·to·my
pan·cre·at·i·co·je·ju·nos·to·my
pan·cre·atin
pan·cre·a·tism
pan·cre·a·tit·ic

pan·cre·a·ti·tis
pan·cre·a·tog·e·nous
pan·cre·at·o·lith
pan·cre·a·to·li·thot·o·my
pan·cre·a·tol·y·sis
pan·cre·a·tot·o·my
pan·cre·op·a·thy
pan·cy·tol·y·sis
pan·cy·to·pe·nia
pan·cy·to·sis
pan·dem·ic
pan·dic·u·la·tion
pan·e·lec·tro·scope
pan·en·do·scope
pan·es·the·sia
pan·es·thet·ic
pang
pan·hi·dro·sis
pan·hy·grous
pan·hys·ter·ec·to·my
pan·hys·ter·o—oo·pho·rec·to·my
pan·hys·ter·o·sal·pin·gec·to·my
pan·ic
pan·im·mu·ni·ty
pa·niv·o·rous
pan·mix·ia or pan·mix·ie
pan·mne·sia
pan·my·e·lop·a·thy
pan·my·e·loph·thi·sis

61

pan·my·e·lo·tox·i-
   co·sis
pan·ni pl.
pan·nic·u·li·tis
pan·nic·u·lus
pan·nus sing.
pano·pho·bia
pan·oph·thal·mi·tis
pan·os·te·i·tis
pan·o·ti·tis
pan·scle·ro·sis
pan·si·nus·i·tis
pant
pan·ta·mor·phia
pan·ta·mor·phic
pan·ta·pho·bia
pan·ta·tro·phia
pan·te·the·ine
pan·to·caine
pan·to·paque
pan·to·pho·bia
pan·to·then·yl
pan·trop·ic
pa·nus
pap
pa·pa·in
pa·pav·er·ine
pa·pes·cent
pa·pil·la sing.
pa·pil·lae pl.
pap·il·lar
pa·pil·la·ry
pa·pil·late
pap·il·lat·ed
pap·il·lec·to·my
pap·il·le·de·ma

pap·il·lif·er·ous
pa·pil·li·form
pap·il·li·tis
pap·il·lo·ma sing.
pap·il·lo·mas or
   pap·il·lo·ma·ta pl.
pap·il·lo·ma·to·sis
pap·il·lo·ma·tous
pa·pil·lo·ret·i·ni·tis
pap·pi pl.
pap·pose
pap·pus sing.
pap·u·lar
pap·u·lat·ed
pap·u·la·tion
pap·ule
pap·u·lif·er·ous
pap·u·lo·pus·tu·lar
pap·u·lose
pap·u·lo·squa·mous
pap·u·lo·ve·sic·u-
   lar
pap·y·ra·ceous
para—an·al·ge·sia
para—an·es·the·sia
para—ap·pen·di·ci-
   tis
para·blep·sia or
   para·blep·sy
para·bu·lia
para·can·tho·ma
para·can·tho·sis
para·cen·te·ses pl.
para·cen·te·sis sing.
para·cen·tral
para·chlor·phe·nol

para·cho·lia
para·chor·dal
para·chro·ma·tism
para·chro·ma·top-
   sia
para·chro·mo·phore
para·chro·mo·phor-
   ic
par·ac·me
para·co·li·tis
para·co·lon
para·col·pi·tis
par·a·col·pi·um
para·con·dy·lar
para·cone
para·co·nid
par·acu·sia or
   par·acu·sis
para·cy·e·sis
para·cys·tic
para·cys·ti·tis
para·cy·tic
para·de·ni·tis
para·den·tal
para·di·ag·no·sis
para·did·y·mis
para·du·o·de·nal
para·dys·en·tery
para·ep·i·lep·sy
par·af·fin
para·gam·ma·cism
para·gan·gli·o·ma
para·gan·gli·on
para·gas·tric
para·gen·i·tal·is
par·a·gen·sia

par·a·gen·sis
par·ag·glu·ti·na-
  tion
para·glos·sa sing.
para·glos·sae pl.
para·glos·sia
pa·rag·na·thous
pa·rag·na·thus
para·gom·pho·sis
par·a·gon·i·mi·a·sis
para·gram·ma·tism
para·graph·ia
para·he·mo·phil·ia
para·he·pat·ic
para·hep·a·ti·tis
para·hor·mone or
  para·hor·mon·ic
para·hyp·no·sis
para·in·flu·en·za
para·ker·a·to·sis
para·ki·ne·sia or
  para·ki·ne·sis
para·la·lia
para·lep·ro·sis
para·le·re·ma
para·le·re·sis
para·lex·ia
par·al·ge·sia
par·al·gia
par·al·lac·tic
par·al·lax
par·al·lel·ism
par·al·lel·om·e·ter
pa·ral·ler·gy
para·lo·gia
pa·ral·o·gism

pa·ral·o·gis·tic
pa·ral·o·gize
pa·ral·y·sis
par·a·lyt·ic
par·a·ly·zant
par·a·ly·za·tion
par·a·lyze
par·a·lyz·er
para·mag·net·ic
para·mag·ne·tism
para·mas·ti·tis
para·mas·toid·i·tis
para·me·di·an
para·me·nia
para·metha·di·one
para·me·tria (sing.:
  parametrium)
para·me·tri·al
para·met·ric
para·met·rism
para·me·tri·tis
para·me·tri·um (pl.:
  parametria)
para·me·trop·a·thy
para·mim·ia
par·am·ne·sia
para·mo·lar
para·mu·cin
para·mu·sia
par·am·y·loid
para·na·sal
para·ne·phri·tis
para·neu·ral
para·noia
para·noi·ac
para·noid

par·an·tral
para·nu·cle·us
para·pan·cre·at·ic
para·per·tus·sis
par·a·pha·sia
para·phil·ia
para·phil·i·ac
para·phi·mo·sis
para·pho·bia
para·pho·nia
para·phra·sia
para·phre·ni·tis
para·plasm
para·plas·tic
para·plec·tic
para·ple·gia
para·ple·gic
para·pneu·mo·nia
pa·rap·o·plexy
para·prax·ia
para·proc·ti·tis
para·proc·tium
para·pros·ta·ti·tis
para·pso·ri·a·sis
para·psy·chol·o·gy
para·rec·tal
para·sa·cral
para·sag·it·tal
para·sal·pin·gi·tis
para·se·cre·tion
para·sex·u·al·i·ty
par·a·site
par·a·sit·ic
par·a·sit·i·cide
par·a·sit·iza·tion
par·a·si·to·gen·ic

par·a·si·tol·o·gy
par·a·sito·pho·bia
par·a·sit·osis
par·a·si·to·trop·ic
para·small·pox
par·a·some
para·spa·di·as
para·spasm
para·ster·nal
para·sym·pa·thet-
ic
para·sym·pa·tho-
lyt·ic
para·syn·ap·sis
para·syph·i·lis
para·te·re·si·o-
ma·nia
para·thy·roid·al
para·thy·roid·ec-
to·my
para·thy·ro·pri·val
para·thy·ro·trop·ic
para·ton·sil·lar
para·tri·cho·sis
para·trip·sis
para·troph·ic
pa·rat·ro·phy
para·typh·li·tis
para·ty·phoid
para·ure·thral
para·u·ter·ine
para·vac·cin·ia
para·vag·i·nal
para·vag·i·ni·tis
para·ver·te·bral
para·ves·i·cal

par·ax·i·al
par·ec·ta·sis *or*
  par·ec·ta·sia
par·e·gor·ic
pa·ren·chy·ma
par·en·chym·a·ti·tis
par·en·chym·a·tous
par·ent
pa·ren·tal
par·en·ter·al
par·ep·i·thym·ia
par·er·ga·sia
pa·re·ses pl.
pa·re·sis sing.
par·es·the·sia
pa·ret·i·cal·ly
pa·reu·nia
par·hi·dro·sis
pa·ri·etal
pa·ri·e·to·fron·tal
pa·ri·e·to—oc·cip-
i·tal
par·kin·son·ism
paro·don·ti·tis
paro·don·ti·um
par·o·nych·ia
par·oph·thal·mia
pa·ro·pia
par·op·sia *or* par-
op·sis
par·o·ra·sis
par·o·rex·ia
par·os·mia
par·os·ti·tis
par·os·to·sis
pa·rotic

par·otid
pa·rot·i·dec·to·my
pa·rot·i·do·scle-
ro·sis
par·o·tit·ic
par·oti·tis
par·ous
par·o·va·ri·ot·o·my
par·o·va·ri·tis
par·o·var·i·um
par·ox·ysm
par·ox·ys·mal
par·rot fe·ver
pars
par·ti·cle n. (small
  part; cf. *pedicle*)
par·tic·u·late
par·ti·tion
par·tu·ri·en·cy
par·tu·ri·ent
par·tu·ri·fa·cient
par·tu·ri·om·e·ter
par·tu·ri·tion
par·tus
pa·ru·lis
par·um·bil·i·cal
par·vi·cel·lu·lar
par·vi·loc·u·lar
par·vule
pas·sage
pas·sion
pas·si·vate
pas·sive
pas·teur·iza·tion
pas·teur·iz·er
pas·tille

pate
pa·tel·la sing.
pa·tel·lae or pa·tel·las pl.
pa·tel·lec·to·my
pa·ten·cy
pa·tent adj.
pat·ent n., v.
path·er·ga·sia
path·er·gy or path·er·gia
pa·thet·ic
path·o·don·tia
patho·gen
patho·gen·e·sis
patho·ge·net·ic
patho·ge·nic·i·ty
patho·log·ic
patho·log·i·cal
pa·thol·o·gist
pa·thol·o·gy
path·o·phor·ic
patho·psy·chol·o·gy
pa·thos
pa·tho·sis
pa·tience
pa·tient
pat·ten
pat·tern
pat·u·lous
paunch
paunchy
pause
pave·ment·ing
pa·vor

pec·tase
pec·ten (body part)
pec·tin (water-soluble substance)
pec·tin·ase
pec·ti·nate
pec·tin·e·al
pec·tin·e·us
pec·to·ral
pec·to·ra·les pl.
pec·to·ra·lis sing.
pec·to·ril·o·quy
pec·tose
pec·tous
pec·tus
ped·er·as·ty
pe·des (sing.: pes)
pe·de·sis
ped·i·al·gia
pe·di·a·tri·cian
pe·di·at·rics
pe·di·a·trist
ped·i·at·ry
ped·i·cel·late
ped·i·cle (slender stem; cf. particle)
pe·dic·te·rus
pe·dic·u·lar
pe·dic·u·la·tion
pe·dic·u·li·cide
pe·dic·u·lo·ses pl.
pe·dic·u·lo·sis sing.
pe·dic·u·lous
ped·i·cure
pe·do·don·tics
pe·do·don·tist

pe·dol·o·gist
pe·dol·o·gy
pe·dom·e·ter
pe·dop·a·thy
pe·do·phil·ia or pae·do·phil·ia
pe·do·pho·bia
pe·dun·cle
pe·dun·cu·lar
pe·dun·cu·late
peel·ing
pel·age
pel·la·gra
pel·la·grin
pel·la·grous
pel·let
pel·le·tier·ine
pel·li·cle
pel·lic·u·la
pel·lic·u·lar
pel·lu·cid
pel·oid
pe·lop·sia
pelo·ther·a·py
pel·vic
pel·vis sing.
pel·vi·sac·ral
pel·vi·scope
pel·vis·es or pel·ves pl.
pem·mi·can
pem·phi·goid
pem·phi·gus
pen·du·lous·ness
pe·nes or pe·nis·es (sing.: penis)

65

pen·e·trat·ing
pen·e·tra·tion
pen·i·cil·li (sing.: *pen-icillus*)
pen·i·cil·lin
pen·i·cil·lin·ase
pen·i·cil·li·um
pen·i·cil·lus (pl.: *penicilli*)
pe·nis (pl.: *penes* or *penises*)
pen·ny·weight
pen·ta·chlo·ro-phe·nol
pen·tad
pen·ta·dac·tyl
pen·ta·quine
pen·ta·stome *or* pen·tas·to·mid *or* pen·tas·to·moid
pen·ta·tom·ic
pen·ta·va·lent
pen·to·bar·bi·tal
pen·to·tom·i
pen·tyl
pe·o·til·lo·ma·nia
pep·per·mint
pep·si·gogue
pep·sin
pep·sin·o·gen
pep·tic
pep·ti·dase
pep·tide
pep·ti·za·tion
pep·to·gen·ic *or* pep·tog·e·nous

pep·tone
pep·to·nize
pep·to·nu·ria
per·a·cid·i·ty
per·acute
per   an·num (yearly)
per·a·num (anally)
per·cent
per·cen·tile
per·cep·tion
per·cep·tiv·i·ty
per·cep·tu·al·ly
per·clu·sion
per·co·la·tion
per·co·la·tor
per·cus·sion
per·cus·sor
per·cu·ta·ne·ous
per·fo·rans
per·fo·rat·ed
per·fo·ra·tion
per·fri·ca·tion
per·fuse
per·fu·sion
peri·ad·e·ni·tis
peri·anal
peri·an·gi·i·tis
peri·aor·ti·tis
peri·ap·i·cal
peri·ar·te·ri·al
peri·ar·te·ri·tis
peri·ar·thri·tis
peri·ar·tic·u·lar
peri·au·ric·u·lar
peri·ax·i·al
peri·blep·sis

peri·bron·chi·al
peri·bron·chi·tis
peri·cap·il·lary
peri·car·dia (sing.: *pericardium*)
peri·car·di·ec·to·my
peri·car·di·os·to·my
peri·car·di·ot·o·my
peri·car·dit·i·des pl.
peri·car·di·tis sing.
peri·car·di·um (pl.: *pericardia*)
peri·carp
peri·car·pi·al
peri·car·pic
peri·ce·cal
peri·ce·men·ti·tis
peri·ce·men·tum
peri·cha·reia
peri·chol·an·gi·tis
peri·chol·e·cys·tic
peri·chol·e·cys·ti·tis
peri·chon·dri·tis
peri·chon·dri·um
peri·chord·al
peri·co·li·tis
peri·cor·ne·al
peri·cor·o·ni·tis
peri·cra·ni·um
peri·cys·tic
peri·cys·ti·tis
peri·cys·ti·um
peri·cyte
peri·cy·tial
peri·den·tal
peri·den·ti·tis

peri·derm
peri·der·mal
peri·der·mic
peri·di·ver·tic·u-
    li·tis
peri·du·ral
peri·en·ceph·a·li·tis
peri·en·ter·ic
peri·ep·en·dy·mal
peri·esoph·a·ge·al
peri·fis·tu·lar
peri·fol·lic·u·li·tis
peri·gan·gli·i·tis
peri·gan·gli·on·ic
peri·la·ryn·ge·al
peri·lymph
peri·lym·phan·ge·al
peri·lym·phan·gi·tis
peri·lym·phat·ic
pe·rim·e·ter
peri·met·ric
peri·me·tri·um
pe·rim·e·try
    (measuring field of
    vision)
pé·rim·i·try
peri·my·e·li·tis
peri·my·o·si·tis
peri·my·sia pl.
peri·my·si·um sing.
peri·na·tal
per·i·ne·al (pertaining
    to perineum; cf. peri-
    toneal, peroneal)
peri·neph·ric

peri·ne·phri·tis
peri·neph·ri·um
per·i·ne·um (area
    bounded by thighs;
    cf. peritoneum)
peri·neu·ral
peri·neu·ri·al
peri·neu·ri·tis
peri·neu·ri·um
peri·nu·cle·ar
peri·oc·u·lar
pe·ri·od
pe·ri·od·ic
pe·ri·od·i·cal·ly
peri·odon·tal
peri·odon·tia pl.
peri·odon·tics
peri·odon·tist
peri·odon·ti·um
    sing.
peri·odon·to·cla·sia
peri·odon·tol·o·gy
peri·odon·to·sis
pe·ri·od·o·scope
peri·o·dyn·ia
peri·om·phal·ic
peri·onych·ia pl.
peri·onych·i·um
    sing.
peri·on·yx
peri·or·al
peri·or·bit
peri·os·te·al
peri·os·te·um
peri·os·ti·tis
peri·os·to·ma

peri·otic
pe·riph·er·al
pe·riph·ery
peri·phle·bi·tis
peri·pla·ne·ta
peri·pleu·ri·tis
peri·por·tal
peri·proc·tal
peri·proc·tic
peri·proc·ti·tis
peri·pro·stat·ic
peri·py·le·phle-
    bi·tis
peri·rec·tal
peri·re·nal
peri·sal·pin·gi·tis
peri·sin·u·ous
peri·splen·ic
peri·sple·ni·tis
peri·stal·sis
peri·stal·tic
peri·sta·sis
peri·stome
per·is·ton
peri·syn·o·vi·al
peri·tec·to·my
peri·ten·din·e·um
peri·ten·di·ni·tis
peri·ten·on
peri·the·li·um
peri·to·ne·al (of
    peritoneum; cf. peri-
    neal, peroneal)
peri·to·neo·scope
peri·to·neo·scop·ic
peri·to·ne·os·co·py

67

peri·to·ne·um
  (serous membrane;
  cf. *perineum*)
peri·to·ni·tis
peri·ton·sil·lar
peri·ton·sil·li·tis
peri·typhl·ic
peri·um·bil·i·cal
peri·un·gual
peri·uter·ine
peri·vas·cu·lar
  (around blood vessel;
  cf. *perivesical*)
peri·ve·ni·tis
peri·ve·nous
peri·ves·i·cal
  (around urinary blad-
  der; cf. *perivascular*)
perle
per·lèche
per·ma·nent·ly
per·me·abil·i·ty
per·me·able
per·me·ation
per·ni·cious
per·ni·o·sis
pero·bra·chi·us
pero·dac·tyl·ia
pe·ro·ne·al
  (pertaining to fibula;
  cf. *perineal, peri-
  toneal*)
per·o·ne·us
per·o·nia
per·oral
per·os

pe·ro·ses pl.
pe·ro·sis sing.
per·ox·ide
per·ox·i·dize
per·pen·dic·u·lar
per primam
per·sev·er·a·tion
per·sim·mon
per·son·al·i·ty
per·spi·ra·tion
per·spire
per·sul·fate
per·tur·ba·tion
per·tus·sal
per·tus·sis
per·vap·o·ra·tion
per·ver·sion
per·vert
per·vi·gil·i·um
per·y·lene
pes (pl.: *pedes*)
pes·sa·ry
pes·su·lus
pes·ti·cide
pes·tis
pes·tle
pe·te·chia sing.
pe·te·chi·ae pl.
pe·tit mal
pet·ri·fac·tion
pe·tris·sage
pet·ro·la·tum
pe·tro·le·um
pe·tro·sa
pe·tro·sal
pe·trous

pe·trox·o·lin
pha·ci·tis
phac·o·er·l·sis
pha·coid
pha·col·y·sis
phac·o·scle·ro·sis
phac·o·scope
phac·o·sco·tas·mus
phag·e·de·na
phag·e·den·ic
phago·cyte
phago·cyt·ize
phago·cy·tose
phago·cy·to·sis
pha·gol·y·sis
phal·a·cro·sis
pha·lan·ge·al (of
  finger or toe bone; cf.
  pharyngeal)
phal·an·gec·to·my
phal·an·gi·tis
pha·lan·gi·za·tion
pha·lanx sing.
pha·lanx·es *or*
  pha·lan·ges pl.
phal·lic
phal·lus
phan·er·o·gen·ic
phan·er·o·ma·nia
phan·tasm
phar·ci·dous
phar·ma·ceu·tic
phar·ma·ceu·ti·cal
phar·ma·cist
phar·ma·cog·no·
  sist

phar·ma·col·o·gist
phar·ma·col·o·gy
phar·ma·co·ther·a·py
phar·ma·cy
pha·ryn·geal (of the pharynx; cf. *pha·langeal*)
phar·yn·gis·mus
phar·yn·gi·tis
pha·ryn·go·glos·sus
pha·ryn·go·log·i·cal
phar·yn·gol·o·gy
phar·yn·gol·y·sis
pha·ryn·go·na·sal
pha·ryn·gor·rhea
pha·ryn·go·scope
pha·ryn·go·spasm
phar·yn·got·o·my
phar·ynx
phase
phat·nor·rha·gia
phe·na·caine *or* phe·no·cain
phen·a·kis·to·scope
phen·an·threne
phe·nate
phen·a·zone
phene
phe·net·i·dine
phe·net·sal
phe·no·bar·bi·tal
pheno·coll
phe·no·copy
phe·nol
phe·no·lase

phe·nom·e·na *or* phe·nom·e·nons pl.
phe·nom·e·non sing.
phe·no·thi·azine
phe·no·type
phe·no·typ·ic
phe·no·typ·i·cal
phe·noxy
phenyl·eph·rine
phenyl·hy·dra·zine
phe·nyl·ic
phenyl·ke·to·nu·ria
pheo·chro·mo·cy·to·ma
pheo·phy·tin *or* phaeo·phy·tin
phi·a·loph·o·ra
phil·ter *or* phil·tre
phil·trum
phi·mo·sis
phi·mot·ic
phle·bec·to·my
phleb·ex·ai·re·sis
phle·bis·mus
phle·bi·tis
phlebo·cly·sis
phleb·o·gram
phleb·o·graph·ic
phle·bog·ra·phy
phleb·oid
phleb·o·lith
phlebo·scle·ro·sis
phlebo·throm·bo·sis
phleb·o·tome
phle·bot·o·my

phlegm
phleg·ma·sia
phleg·mat·ic
phleg·mat·i·cal
phleg·mon·ous
phlog·o·gen·ic
phlor·e·tin
phlor·i·zin
phlor·o·glu·cin·ol
phylc·te·na *or* phylc·tae·na
phlyc·ten·ule
pho·bia
pho·bic
pho·com·e·lus
pho·nal
phon·as·the·nia
pho·na·tion
pho·neme
pho·net·ics
pho·nics
pho·no·car·di·o·graph
pho·no·pho·bia
pho·rop·tor
phose
phos·pha·tase
phos·phate
phos·pha·te·mia
phos·phene (sensation)
phos·phine (gas)
phos·pho·res·cent
phos·pho·ric
phos·pho·rous
pho·tic

pho·tism
pho·to·ca·tal·y·sis
pho·to·elec·tric
pho·to·elec·tron
pho·tom·e·ter
pho·ton·o·sus
pho·to·sen·si·ti·za-
tion
pho·to·syn·the·sis
phren·as·the·nia
phre·nic
phren·i·cec·to·my
phren·i·cot·o·my
phren·o·car·dia
phren·o·car·di·ac
phren·o·ple·gia
phren·o·sin
phro·ne·sis
phry·no·der·ma
phthal·ate
phthi·ri·a·sis
phthir·i·us
phthis·i·ol·o·gy
phygo·ga·lac·tic
phy·lax·is
phy·log·e·ny
phy·ma
phy·ma·to·sis
phys·i·an·thro·py
phys·iat·rics
phys·i·at·rist
phys·ic
phys·i·cal
phy·si·cian
phys·i·co·chem·i·
cal

phys·i·co·gen·ic
phys·i·og·no·my
phys·i·o·log·ic
phys·i·o·log·i·cal·ly
phys·i·ol·o·gist
phys·i·ol·o·gy
phy·sique
phy·so·stig·mine
phy·tol
phy·to·sis
pia ma·ter
pi·ce·ous
pic·ro·car·mine
pic·ro·tox·in
pie·dra
pi·es·es·the·sia
pi·geon—toed
pig·men·ta·tion
pig·men·to·phage
pi·lar
pi·la·ry
pi·las·tered
pi·le·o·us
piles
pi·li·a·tion
pi·li·gan
pil·lar
pil·let
pi·lo·car·pine
pi·lo·car·pus
pi·lo·cys·tic
pi·lo·mo·tor
pi·lo·ni·dal
pi·lose
pi·lo·se·ba·ceous
pi·lo·sis

pi·los·i·ty
pil·u·lar or pil·lu·lar
pi·lus
pi·men·ta
pim·ple
pin·a·cy·a·nol
pince·ment
pi·ne·al
pin·e·a·lo·ma
pin·guid
pink·eye
pin·na
pi·on
pi·or·thop·nea
pi·pette
pir·i·for·mis or
pyr·i·for·mis
pis·cid·ia
pi·si·form
pith·i·a·tism
pit·ted
pit·ting
pi·tu·itary
pit·y·ri·a·sis
piv·ot·ing
pla·ce·bo
pla·cen·ta
pla·cen·ta·tion
plac·en·ti·tis
plac·en·tog·ra·phy
plac·en·to·ma
plac·ode
pla·gi·o·ceph·a·ly
plague
plane
pla·ni·ceps

plank·ton
pla·no—con·cave
pla·no—con·vex
plan·tar
plan·tar·is
plan·ta·tion
plan·ti·grade
pla·num
plaque
plas·ma
plas·ma·cyte
plas·ma·cy·to·sis
plas·ma·lem·ma
plas·mat·ic
plas·mic
plas·mi·cal·ly
plas·min
plas·min·o·gen
plas·mo·cy·to·ma
plas·mo·di·um
plas·mog·a·my
plas·ter
plas·tic
plas·tic·i·ty
pla·teau
plate·let
platy·ce·lous *or*
  platy·coe·lous
platy·ce·phal·ic
platy·mer·ic
platy·pel·lic
plat·yr·rhine
pla·tys·ma
pled·get
plei·ot·ro·pism
ple·o·chro·ic

ple·och·ro·ism
ple·o·cy·to·sis
pleo·mor·phism
ple·o·nex·ia
ple·ro·sis
pleth·o·ra
ple·thys·mo·graph
pleu·ra sing.
pleu·rae *or* pleu·
  ras pl.
pleu·ral
pleur·apoph·y·sis
pleu·ri·sy
pleu·rit·ic
pleu·ro·dyn·ia
pleu·ro·gen·ic
pleu·ro·pneu·mo·nia
pleu·ro·pul·mo·nary
plex·im·e·ter
plex·or
plex·us
pli·ca
pli·cate
pli·ca·tion
plomb
plom·bage
plug·ger
plum·ba·gin
plum·bism
plu·ri·glan·du·lar
plu·ri·grav·i·da
plu·rip·a·ra
plu·to·ni·um
pne·o·dy·nam·ics
pneu·ma·ti·za·tion
pneu·ma·to·cele

pneu·ma·tom·e·ter
pneu·ma·to·sis
pneu·mo·ba·cil·lus
pneu·mo·cen·te·sis
pneu·mo·coc·cal
pneu·mo·coc·ce·mia
pneu·mo·coc·cus
pneu·mo·co·ni·o·sis
pneu·mo·en·ceph·a·
  lo·gram
pneu·mo·en·ter·i·tis
pneu·mo·gas·tric
pneu·mog·ra·phy
pneu·mo·me·di·as·
  ti·num
pneu·mo·nia
pneu·mon·ic
pneu·mo·ni·tis
pneu·mo·nol·y·sis
pneu·mo·nop·a·thy
pneu·mo·not·o·my
pneu·mo·per·i·car·
  di·tis
pneu·mo·per·i·car·
  di·um
pneu·mo·per·i·to·
  ne·um
pneu·mo·tho·rax
pneu·sis
pock
pock·mark n., v.
po·dag·ra
po·dal·ic
pod·e·de·ma
po·di·a·trist
po·di·a·try

podo·brom·hi·dro-
sis
podo·dyn·ia
po·go·ni·on
poi·kilo·blast
poi·kilo·cy·to·sis
poi·kilo·der·ma
poise
poi·son ivy
poi·son·ous
po·lar·i·ty
po·lar·iza·tion
po·lar·ize
po·lar·iz·er
po·lar·og·ra·phy
po·lio·en·ceph·a-
li·tis
po·lio·my·eli·tis
po·lio·my·e·lop·a-
thy
po·li·o·sis
pol·len
pol·le·no·sis
pol·lex
pol·lu·tion
po·lo·cyte
pol·toph·a·gy
po·lus
poly·an·dry
poly·ar·thri·tis
poly·ar·tic·u·lar
poly·cel·lu·lar
poly·cen·tric
poly·clin·ic
poly·cy·e·sis
poly·cy·the·mia

poly·dip·sia
poly·ga·lac·tia
poly·mer
po·ly·mer·iza·tion
poly·mor·pho·nu-
cle·ar
poly·my·o·si·tis
poly·myx·in
poly·neu·ri·tis
poly·odon·tia
poly·o·pia
poly·o·rex·ia
pol·yp
poly·pa·re·sis
poly·pha·gia
poly·pho·bia
poly·pnea
pol·yp·oid
poly·po·rous
pol·yp·o·sis
poly·se·ro·si·tis
poly·so·mic
poly·sper·my
poly·tro·phic
poly·uria
pom·pho·ly·he·mia
pom·pho·lyx
pon·der·a·ble
pons sing.
pon·tes pl.
pon·tic
pon·to·caine
pop·li·te·al
pop·lit·e·us
pore
po·ro·sis

po·ros·i·ty
po·rous
por·phyr·ia
por·poise
por·ta
por·ta·ca·val
por·tal
por·tio
po·rus
po·si·tion
pos·i·tive
po·sol·o·gy
post·a·nal
post·ap·o·plec·tic
post·ax·i·al
post·ca·va
post·cla·vic·u·lar
post·co·i·tal
post·em·bry·on·ic
post·en·ceph·a·lit·ic
post·ep·i·lep·tic
pos·te·ri·ad
pos·te·ri·or
pos·tero·an·te·ri·or
pos·tero·ex·ter·nal
pos·tero·in·ter·nal
pos·tero·lat·er·al
pos·tero·me·di·al
pos·tero·su·pe·ri·or
post·fe·brile
pos·thi·tis
post·hu·mous
post·hyp·not·ic
post·mor·tem
post·na·sal
post·na·tal

post·oc·u·lar
post·op·er·a·tive
post·oral
post·pran·di·al
post·trau·mat·ic
pos·tu·late
pos·tur·al
pos·ture
po·ta·bil·i·ty
po·ta·ble
pot·ash
po·tas·si·um
po·ten·cy
po·ten·tial
po·ten·ti·a·tion
po·tion
pouch
poul·tice
pow·der
pox
prac·tice
prag·mat·ag·no·sia
prag·mat·am·ne·sia
prag·mat·ic
pran·di·al
pre·anal
pre·an·es·thet·ic
pre·an·ti·sep·tic
pre·ax·i·al
pre·can·cer·ous
pre·ca·va
pre·cip·i·tant
pre·cip·i·tate
pre·cip·i·ta·tion
pre·cip·i·ta·tor
pre·clin·i·cal

pre·co·cious
pre·coc·i·ty
pre·cog·ni·tion
pre·con·vul·sant
pre·con·vul·sive
pre·cor·di·um
pre·cos·tal
pre·cu·ne·us
pre·di·gest·ed
pre·di·ges·tion
pre·dis·pos·ing
pre·dis·po·si·tion
pre·dor·mi·tion
pre·ec·lamp·sia
pre·for·ma·tive
pre·fron·tal
preg·nan·cy
preg·nant
pre·hen·sion
pre·lo·co·mo·tion
pre·lum
pre·ma·ture
pre·max·il·la
pre·med·i·ca·tion
pre·men·stru·al
pre·mo·lar
pre·mo·ni·tion
pre·mon·i·to·ri·ly
pre·mon·i·to·ry
pre·mu·ni·tion
pre·na·tal
pre·oc·cip·i·tal
prep·a·ra·tion
pre·pa·tel·lar
pre·pat·ent
pre·pon·der·ance

pre·po·ten·cy
pre·po·tent
pre·psy·chot·ic
pre·pu·ber·al
pre·pu·bes·cent
pre·puce
pre·pu·cot·o·my
pre·pu·tial
pre·py·lor·ic
pre·rec·tal
pre·re·nal
pre·re·pro·duc·tive
pre·ret·i·nal
pres·by·at·rics
pres·by·cu·sis
pres·by·der·ma
pres·by·opia
pres·by·opic
pre·scribe
pre·scrip·tion
pre·se·nil·i·ty
pres·ent adj., n.
pre·sent v.
pre·sen·ta·tion
pres·sor adj.
pres·so·re·cep·tor
pres·sure
pre·sys·to·le
pre·sys·tol·ic
prev·a·lence
pre·ven·tive
pre·ven·to·ri·um
pre·ver·tig·i·nous
pre·ves·i·cal
pre·zo·nu·lar
pri·a·pism

prick·ly
pri·ma·ry
pri·mate
pri·mi·grav·i·da
pri·mip·a·ra
pri·mip·a·rous
pri·mi·ti·ae
prim·i·tive
pri·mor·di·al
pri·mor·di·um
prin·ceps
prin·ci·pal adj., n. (head)
prin·ci·ple n. (rule)
prism
pris·mat·ic
pris·moid
pro·am·ni·on
pro·bang
probe
pro·bos·cis
pro·caine
pro·cal·lus
pro·ce·dure
proc·er·us
pro·cess
pro·ces·sus
proci·den·tia
pro·cre·ate
pro·cre·a·tion
proct·al·gia
proc·ti·tis
proc·to·cly·sis
proc·to·dae·um
proc·to·log·ic
proc·tol·o·gist

proc·to·scope
proc·to·scop·ic
proc·tos·co·py
proc·tos·to·my
pro·cum·bent
pro·cur·va·tion
pro·dig·i·o·sin
pro·dro·mal
pro·drome
prod·uct
pro·duc·tive
pro·en·zyme
pro·fes·sion·al
pro·fla·vine
pro·fun·da pl.
pro·fun·dus sing.
pro·gen·er·ate
pro·gen·i·tor
prog·e·ny
pro·ge·ria
pro·ges·ter·one
prog·na·thic
prog·na·thism
prog·no·ses pl.
prog·no·sis sing.
prog·nos·tic
prog·nos·ti·cate
prog·nos·ti·cian
pro·grav·id
pro·gres·sive
pro·i·o·tia
pro·jec·tion
pro·la·bi·um
pro·lac·tin
pro·la·min or pro·la·mine

pro·lapse
pro·lap·sus
pro·lep·sis
pro·lif·er·ate
pro·lif·er·a·tion
pro·lif·ic
pro·lig·er·ous
pro·line
pro·me·thi·um
pro·min
prom·i·nence
promi·zole
pro·mon·o·cyte
prom·on·to·ry
pro·my·e·lo·cyte
pro·nate
pro·na·tion
pro·na·tor
prone
pro·neph·ros
prong
pro·nu·cle·us
pro·otic
pro·pae·deu·tic
prop·a·gate
prop·a·ga·tion
pro·pam·i·dine
pro·pane
pro·per·din
pro·per·i·to·ne·al
pro·phase
pro·phy·lac·tic
pro·phy·lax·is
pro·pi·o·nate
pro·pos·i·tus
pro·pri·etary

pro·prio·cep·tion
pro·prio·cep·tive
pro·prio·cep·tor
pro·pri·us
pro·pto·sis
pro·pul·sion
pro·pyl
pro·re·na·ta
pro·sec·tor
pros·o·cele *or*
  pros·o·coele
pros·o·dem·ic
pro·sop·ic
pros·tate
pros·ta·tec·to·my
pros·ta·tism
pros·ta·ti·tis
pros·ta·to·cys·ti·tis
pros·tat·o·gram
pros·ta·tog·ra·phy
pros·tat·o·lith
pros·ta·tor·rhea
pros·ta·tot·o·my
pro·ster·num
pros·the·sis
pros·thet·ics
pros·the·tist
pros·thi·on
pros·tho·don·tia
prosth·odon·tist
pro·stig·min·ine *or*
  pro·stig·mine
pros·ti·tu·tion
pros·trate .
prot·amine
pro·ta·no·pia

pro·te·an adj.
  (able to change form;
  cf. *protein*)
pro·te·ase
pro·tec·tive
pro·te·i·form
pro·tein n.
  (nitrogenous com-
  pounds; cf. *protean*)
pro·tein·ase
pro·tein·e·mia
pro·tein·uria
pro·te·ol·y·sis
pro·te·ose
pro·throm·bin
pro·thy·mia
pro·ti·um
pro·to·blast
pro·to·blas·tic
pro·to·cone
pro·to·co·nid
pro·to·gen
pro·to·path·ic
pro·to·pla·sis
pro·to·plasm
pro·to·plas·mat·ic
pro·to·plas·mic
pro·to·plast
pro·to·pro·te·ose
pro·to·spasm
pro·to·tro·phic
pro·tot·ro·py
pro·to·ver·a·trine
pro·to·ver·te·bra
pro·to·zoa pl.
pro·to·zo·a·cide

pro·to·zo·an
pro·to·zo·i·a·sis
pro·to·zo·ol·o·gist
pro·to·zo·on sing.
pro·tract
pro·trac·tor
pro·trude
pro·tru·sion
pro·tu·ber·ance
proud flesh
pro·vi·ta·min
pro·voc·a·tive
prox·i·mal
prox·i·mate
prox·i·mo·a·tax·ia
prox·i·mo·buc·cal
pro·zone
pru·i·nate
pru·ri·go
pru·rit·ic
pru·ri·tus
prus·si·ate
prus·sic
psam·mo·ma
psam·mous
psel·lism
psel·lis·mus
pseu·des·the·sia
pseu·di·a·ter
pseu·do·ath·er·o·
  ma
pseu·do·blep·sia
pseu·do·bulb·ar
pseu·do·car·ti·lage
pseu·do·cir·rho·sis
pseu·do·cy·e·sis

pseu·do·cyst
pseu·do·e·de·ma
pseu·do·hal·lu·ci·na·tion
pseu·do·her·maph·ro·dit·ism
pseu·do·hy·per·troph·ic
pseu·do·hy·per·tro·phy
pseu·do·ma·nia
pseu·dom·o·nas
pseu·do·mor·phine
pseu·do·neu·ri·tis
pseu·do·pa·ral·y·sis
pseu·do·par·a·site
pseu·do·po·di·um
pseu·dop·sia
pseu·dop·to·sis
pseu·do·re·ac·tion
pseu·do·rhon·cus
psi·caine
psit·ta·co·sis
pso·as
pso·i·tis
pso·mo·pha·gia
pso·ra
pso·ri·a·sis
pso·ri·at·ic
psy·cha·gogy
psy·chal·gia
psych·as·the·nia
psy·che
psy·chen·to·nia
psy·chi·a·ter
psy·chi·at·ric

psy·chi·a·trist
psy·chi·a·try
psy·chic
psy·cho·anal·y·sis
psy·cho·an·a·lyst
psy·cho·bi·ol·o·gy
psy·cho·di·ag·nos·tics
psy·cho·dy·nam·ics
psy·cho·gal·va·nom·e·ter
psy·cho·gen·e·sis
psy·cho·gram
psy·cho·graph·ic
psy·cho·ki·ne·sia
psy·cho·ki·ne·sis
psy·cho·lag·ny
psy·cho·lep·sy
psy·cho·log·i·cal·ly
psy·chol·o·gist
psy·chol·o·gy
psy·chom·e·try
psy·cho·mo·tor
psy·cho·neu·ro·log·ic
psy·cho·neu·ro·sis
psy·cho·neu·rot·ic
psy·cho·nom·ics
psy·chon·o·my
psy·cho·path·ia
psy·cho·path·ic
psy·chop·a·thist
psy·cho·patho·log·i·cal
psy·cho·pa·thol·o·gist

psy·cho·pa·thol·o·gy
psy·chop·a·thy
psy·cho·phys·ics
psy·cho·phys·i·o·log·ic
psy·cho·phys·i·ol·o·gy
psy·cho·sen·so·ry
psy·cho·sex·u·al
psy·cho·sis (disorder of mind; cf. *sycosis*)
psy·cho·so·mat·ic
psy·cho·sur·gery
psy·cho·ther·a·py
psy·chot·ic
psy·chro·es·the·sia
psy·chro·lu·sia
psy·chrom·e·ter
psy·chro·phore
psy·chro·ther·a·py
ptar·mic
ptar·mus
pteri·on
pte·ryg·i·um
pter·y·goid
pti·lo·sis
pto·maine
ptosed
pto·sis
ptot·ic
pty·a·lism
pty·a·lo·gen·ic
pty·al·a·gogue
pty·a·lor·rhea
ptys·ma

pu·ber·tal
pu·ber·tas
pu·ber·ty
pu·bes (pl. of *pubis*;
  also, body hair; cf.
  pubis)
pu·bes·cence
pu·bic
pu·bis (sing. of *pubes*;
  also, bones of pelvis;
  cf. *pubes*)
pu·bo·fem·o·ral
pu·bo·pro·stat·ic
pu·den·da pl.
pu·den·dum sing.
pu·er·il·ism
pu·er·i·tia
pu·er·per·al
pu·er·pe·ria pl.
pu·er·pe·ri·um sing.
pu·lex
pu·lic·i·dae
pu·li·cide
pul·lu·late
pul·lu·la·tion
pul·mo·nary
pul·mo·tor
pul·pa·tion
pulp·ec·to·my
pulp·ify
pulp·i·tis
pulp·ot·o·my
pulpy
pul·sate
pul·sa·tile
pul·sa·til·la

pul·sa·tion
pul·sa·tor
pulse·less
pul·sim·e·ter
pul·sus
pul·ta·ceous
pul·ver·ize
pum·ice
punc·tat·ed
punc·tic·u·lum
punc·ti·form
punc·tum
punc·ture
pun·gent
pu·pil
pu·pil·la
pu·pil·lary
pu·pil·lom·e·ter
pu·pil·lo·sta·tom-
  e·ter
pur·ga·tion
pur·ga·tive
purge
pu·ri·fied
pu·ri·form
pu·rine
pu·ri·ty
pu·ro·mu·cous
pur·pu·ra
pur·pu·rin
pu·ru·lence
pu·ru·lent
pu·ru·loid
pu·ru·pu·ru
pus
pus·tu·lant

pus·tu·la·tion
pus·tule
pus·tu·li·form
pus·tu·lo·sis
pus·tu·lous
pu·ta·men
pu·tre·fac·tion
pu·tre·fac·tive
pu·tre·fy
pu·tres·cent
pu·tres·cine
pu·trid
py·ar·thro·sis
pyc·nom·e·ter
pyc·no·phra·sia
pyc·no·sis *or* pyk-
  no·sis
py·el·ec·ta·sia
py·eli·tis
py·elo·gram
py·elog·ra·phy
py·elo·ne·phri·tis
py·el·os·to·my
py·elo·ve·nous
py·emia
py·gal·gia
pyg·my
py·gop·a·gus
pyk·nic
pyk·no·lep·sy
py·le·phle·bi·tis
py·lo·no·plas·ty
py·lo·ric
py·lor·i·tis
py·lo·ro·ste·no·sis
py·lo·rus

77

pyo·cele
pyo·coc·cus
pyo·cy·a·nase
pyo·cy·an·ic
pyo·cy·a·nin
pyo·cyst
pyo·der·ma
pyo·der·ma·to·sis
py·og·e·nes
pyo·gen·e·sis
pyo·gen·ic
py·oid
pyo·me·tra
pyo·ne·phri·tis
pyo·ne·phro·sis
pyo·ne·phrot·ic
pyo·pneu·mo·tho·rax
pyo·poi·e·sis
py·or·rhea
py·o·sis
pyo·sol·pinx
pyo·tho·rax
py·ram·i·da·lis
py·ram·i·dot·o·my
py·ran
pyra·nose
pyr·azine
pyr·azole
py·raz·o·lone
py·rec·tic
py·rene
py·re·nin
py·re·thrum
py·ret·ic
pyr·e·to·gen·ic

pyr·e·tog·e·nous
pyr·e·to·ther·a·py
py·rex·ia
py·rid·azine
pyr·i·dine
pyr·i·form
py·ro·gal·lol
py·ro·gen
py·ro·gen·ic
py·ro·glos·sia
py·ro·lig·ne·ous
py·rol·y·sis
py·ro·ma·nia
py·rom·e·ter
py·rone
py·ro·nine
py·ro·pho·bia
py·ro·punc·ture
py·ro·tax·in
py·rot·ic
py·rox·y·lin
py·uria

quack·ery
qua·dran·gu·lar
quad·rant
quad·ran·ta·no·pia

quad·rate
qua·dra·tus
quad·ri·ceps
quad·ri·cus·pid
quad·rip·a·ra
quad·ri·par·i·ty
qua·drip·a·rous
quad·ri·ple·gia
quad·ri·va·lent
qua·dru·plet
qua·lim·e·ter
qual·i·ta·tive
qual·i·ty
quan·tim·e·ter
quan·ti·ta·tive
quan·tum
quar·an·tine
quar·tan
quar·tip·a·ra
quar·tip·a·rous
qua·ter·na·ry
quer·ce·tin
quick·en·ing
quick·lime
quick·sil·ver
quil·la·ja
quin·a·crine
quin·al·bar·bi·tone
quin·al·dine
quin·al·iz·a·rin
qui·nam·i·dine
quin·i·dine
qui·nine
qui·nin·ism
quin·in·o·der·ma
quin·o·line

qui·none
qui·nox·a·line
quin·que·tu·ber·cu·lar
quin·sy
quin·tan
quin·tip·a·ra
quin·tu·plet
quo·tid·i·an
quo·tient

R

ra·bi·ate
ra·bid
ra·bies
ra·ce·mi·za·tion
ra·ce·mose
ra·chi·cele
ra·chi·cen·te·sis
ra·chil·y·sis
ra·chi·o·camp·sis
ra·chi·o·dyn·ia
ra·chi·o·ple·gia
ra·chi·o·sco·li·o·sis
ra·chi·o·tome
ra·chi·ot·o·my
ra·chip·a·gus
ra·chis
ra·chis·chi·sis

ra·chit·ic
ra·chi·tis
ra·chi·tism
rach·i·to·gen·ic
ra·clage
ra·cle·ment
ra·dec·to·my
ra·di·al
ra·di·a·lis
ra·di·an
ra·di·ant
ra·di·a·tion
rad·i·cal adj. (reaching root or origin)
rad·i·cle n. (root of nerve)
ra·dic·u·lar
ra·dic·u·lec·to·my
ra·dic·u·li·tis
ra·dic·u·lop·a·thy
ra·dii (sing.: *radius*)
ra·dio·ac·tive
ra·dio·ac·tiv·i·ty
ra·dio·co·balt
ra·dio·col·loid
ra·di·o·cur·a·bil·i·ty
ra·di·o·cys·ti·tis
ra·di·ode
ra·di·o·di·ag·no·sis
ra·di·odon·tia
ra·di·odon·tist
ra·dio·gen·ic
ra·di·o·gold
ra·dio·graph
ra·di·og·ra·phy

ra·dio·hu·mer·al
ra·dio·io·dine
ra·dio·iron
ra·dio·iso·tope
ra·di·ol·o·gist
ra·di·ol·o·gy
ra·dio·lu·cent
ra·dio·lu·mi·nes·cence
ra·di·o·mag·ne·si·um
ra·di·on
ra·dio·ne·cro·sis
ra·dio·phos·pho·rus
ra·di·o·prax·is
ra·di·o·re·sist·ance
ra·dio·so·di·um
ra·dio·stron·tium
ra·dio·ther·a·py
ra·dio·ther·my
ra·di·o·tox·e·mia
ra·di·o·trans·par·ent
ra·di·um
ra·di·us (pl.: *radii*)
ra·dix
ra·don
rag·weed
rale
ram·i·fi·ca·tion
ram·i·fy
ram·i·sec·tion
ra·mose
ra·mous
ram·u·lose *or* ram·u·lous

ra·mus
ran·cid·i·ty
ran·u·la
ra·phe
rar·efac·tion
rar·efy
ras·pa·to·ry
ra·tio
ra·tion
ra·tio·nal
rats·bane
rat·tle
re·ac·tion
re·ac·ti·vate
re·ac·ti·va·tion
re·agin
re·al·gar
ream·er
re·am·pu·ta·tion
re·an·i·mate
re·bound
re·cal·ci·fi·ca·tion
re·cal·ci·fied
re·ceiv·er
re·cep·tac·u·lum
re·cep·tive
re·cep·tor
re·cess
re·ces·sion
re·ces·sive
re·cid·i·va·tion
re·cid·i·vism
re·cid·i·vist
rec·i·div·i·ty
rec·i·pe
rec·li·na·tion

re·com·pres·sion
re·con·stit·u·ent
re·con·sti·tu·tion
re·con·struc·tion
re·cov·ery
rec·re·ment
re·cru·des·cence
re·cruit·ment
rec·tal
rec·tal·gia
rec·ti·fi·ca·tion
rec·to·cele
rec·toc·ly·sis
rec·to·coc·cyg·e·al
rec·to·gen·i·tal
rec·to·scope
rec·to·u·re·thra·lis
rec·to·u·ter·ine
rec·to·vag·i·no-
  ab·dom·i·nal
rec·to·ves·i·ca·lis
rec·tum
rec·tus
re·cum·ben·cy
re·cum·bent
re·cu·per·a·tion
re·cu·per·a·tive
re·cur·rence
re·cur·rent
re·cur·va·tion
red·in·te·gra·tion
re·dress·ment
re·duced
re·duc·ible
re·duc·tant
re·duc·tion

re·du·pli·cat·ed
re·du·pli·ca·tion
re·ed·u·ca·tion
re·evo·lu·tion
re·fec·tion
re·flect·ed
re·flec·tion
re·flec·tor
re·flex
re·frac·tive
re·frac·tiv·i·ty
re·frac·tom·e·ter
re·frac·to·ry
re·frac·ture
re·fran·gi·bil·i·ty
re·fresh
re·frig·er·ant
re·frig·er·a·tion
re·fuse v.
ref·use n.
re·fu·sion
re·gen·er·ate
re·gen·er·a·tion
reg·i·men
re·gion
reg·is·ter
reg·is·trar
reg·is·tra·tion
reg·is·try
reg·le·men·ta·tion
re·gres·sion
re·gres·sive
reg·u·lar
reg·u·la·tion
reg·u·la·tive
re·gur·gi·tant

re·gur·gi·ta·tion
re·ha·bil·i·ta·tion
re·ha·la·tion
re·im·plan·ta·tion
re·in·fec·tion
re·in·force·ment
re·in·fu·sion
re·in·ner·va·tion
re·in·oc·u·la·tion
re·in·te·gra·tion
re·in·ver·sion
re·ju·ve·nes·cence
re·lapse
re·la·tion
re·lax·ant
re·lax·ation
re·lief
re·lieve
re·me·di·al
rem·e·dy
re·mis·sion
re·mit·tance
ren
re·nal
re·nes
re·ni·form
re·nin
ren·o·va·tion
re·or·ga·ni·za·tion
re·pel·lent
re·per·cus·sion
re·place·ment
re·plan·ta·tion
re·ple·tion
rep·li·ca·tion
re·po·si·tion

re·pous·soir
re·pres·sion
re·pro·duc·tive
re·pul·sion
re·sect
re·sec·tion
re·sec·to·scope
re·ser·pine
re·serve
res·i·dent
re·sid·u·al
res·i·due
re·sil·ience
re·sil·ient
res·in·oid
re·sis·tance
res·o·lu·tion
re·sol·vent
res·o·nance
res·o·nant
res·o·na·tor
re·sorb·ent
res·or·cin·ol
re·sorp·tion
re·spi·ra·ble
res·pi·ra·tion
res·pi·ra·tor
re·spire
re·sponse
re·spon·si·bil·i·ty
res·ti·tu·tion
res·to·ra·tion
re·stor·ative
re·straint
re·stric·tion
re·strin·gent

re·sul·tant
re·su·pi·nate
re·sus·ci·tate
re·sus·ci·ta·tion
re·sus·ci·ta·tor
re·su·ture
re·tar·dant
re·tard·er
retch
re·te sing.
re·ten·tion
re·tia pl.
re·tic·u·lar
re·tic·u·lat·ed
re·tic·u·lum
re·ti·form
ret·i·na
ret·i·nac·u·lum
ret·i·nal
ret·i·ni·tis
ret·i·nop·a·thy
ret·i·nos·co·py
re·tract
re·trac·til·i·ty
re·trac·tion
re·tro·ac·tion
ret·ro·bul·bar
ret·ro·car·di·ac
ret·ro·ce·cal or
  ret·ro·cae·cal
ret·ro·col·ic
ret·ro·de·vi·a·tion
ret·ro·dis·place-
  ment
ret·ro·e·so·phag-
  e·al

ret·ro·flex·ion *or*
  ret·ro·flec·tion
ret·ro·grade
ret·ro·jec·tion
ret·ro·len·tal
re·tro·lin·gual
ret·ro·mor·pho·sis
ret·ro·na·sal
re·tro·per·i·to·ne·al
ret·ro·phar·ynx
ret·ro·pla·sia
ret·ro·posed
ret·ro·po·si·tion
ret·ro·pul·sion
ret·ro·tra·che·al
ret·ro·vert·ed
re·trude
re·tru·sion
re·union
re·ver·ber·a·tion
rev·er·ie *or* rev·
  ery
re·ver·sal
re·verse
re·ver·sion
re·vi·tal·iza·tion
re·vive
re·viv·i·fi·ca·tion
rev·o·lute
re·vul·sant
re·vul·sive
rhab·do·pho·bia
rha·cous
rhag·a·des
rha·gad·i·form
rhag·oid

rhe
rhe·bo·sce·lia
rhe·bo·sce·lic
rheg·ma
rhem·bas·mus
rheo·base
rhe·o·cord
rhe·om·e·ter
rhe·o·nome
rhe·o·phore
rhe·o·scope
rheo·taxis
rheu·mat·ic
rheu·ma·tism
rheu·ma·toid
rheu·ma·tol·o·gy
rhex·es pl.
rhex·is sing.
rhic·no·sis
rhi·nal
rhi·nal·gia
rhi·nan·tral·gia
rhi·nel·cos
rhi·nism
rhi·ni·tis
rhi·no·by·on
rhi·no·clei·sis
rhi·noc·nes·mus
rhi·no·dyn·ia
rhi·no·ky·pho·sis
rhi·nol·o·gist
rhi·no·mi·o·sis
rhi·nop·a·thy
rhi·no·pho·nia
rhi·no·phyma
rhi·no·pol·yp

rhi·nop·sia
rhi·nor·rha·gia
rhi·nor·rhea *or*
  rhi·nor·rhoea
rhi·no·scope
rhi·nos·co·py
rhi·no·thrix
rhi·not·o·my
rhi·zo·don·tro·py
rhi·zo·mel·ic
rhi·zo·neure
rhi·zot·o·my
rhom·boi·de·us
rhon·chi pl.
rhon·chus sing.
rho·ta·cism
rhy·se·ma
rhythm
rhyth·mic
rhyt·i·do·plas·ty
rhyt·i·do·sis
ri·bo·fla·vin
rick·ets
ri·gid·i·tas
rig·or mor·tis
ri·ma sing.
ri·mae pl.
ring·worm
ri·so·ri·us
ri·sus
ro·den·ti·cide
roent·gen·o·gram
roent·gen·og·ra·phy
roent·gen·ol·o·gist
roent·gen·ol·o·gy
roent·gen·o·lu·cent

roent·gen·o·paque
roent·gen·os·co·py
roent·gen·o·ther·a·py
ron·geur
ro·sa·lia
ro·se·o·la
ro·se·o·lous
ro·sette
ros·in
ros·trum
ro·tat·ing
ro·ta·tion
ro·ta·to·res
rough·age
ru·be·do
ru·be·fa·cient
ru·be·fac·tion
ru·bel·la
ru·be·o·lin
ru·bes·cence
ru·big·i·nous
ru·bor
ruc·ta·tion
ruc·tus
ru·di·men·ta·ry
ru·di·men·tum
ru·fous
ru·ga sing.
ru·gae pl.
ru·gi·tus
ru·gose
ru·gos·i·ty
rum·bling
ru·men sing.
ru·men·ot·o·my

ru·mi·na *or* ru·mens pl.
ru·pia
rup·tio
rup·ture

sab·u·lous
sac
sac·cha·rase
sac·cha·rat·ed
sac·cha·ride
sac·char·i·fi·ca·tion
sac·cha·rim·e·try
sac·cha·rin
sac·cha·ro·my·ces
sac·cha·ro·my·ce·tic
sac·cha·rose
sac·cha·rum
sac·ci·form
sac·cu·lar
sac·cu·lat·ed
sac·cu·la·tion
sac·cule
sac·cu·lus
sac·cus
sa·cra (sing.: *sacrum*)

sa·cral
sac·ral·iza·tion
sac·rec·to·my
sac·ro·coc·cyg·e·us
sa·cro·il·i·ac
sacro·lum·ba·lis
sacro·lum·bar
sacro·pos·te·ri·or
sacro·sci·at·ic
sacro·spi·na·lis
sa·crum (pl.: *sacra*)
sa·dism
sa·dis·tic
sage femme
sa·git·tal
sal
sa·la·cious
sa·lac·i·ty
sal·era·tus
sal·i·cyl·ic
sal·i·cyl·ism
sa·lim·e·ter
sa·line
sa·li·va
sal·i·vant
sal·i·vary
sal·i·va·tion
sa·li·vous
sal·mo·nel·la
sal·mo·nel·lo·sis
sal·pin·gec·to·my
sal·pin·gi·tis
sal·pin·go·cele
sal·pin·go·cy·e·sis
sal·pin·go·pexy
sal·pin·gor·rha·phy

sal·pin·gos·to·my
sal·pin·gys·ter·o-
   cy·e·sis
sal·pinx
sal·ta·tion
sal·ta·to·ry
salt·pe·ter
sa·lu·bri·ous
sa·lu·bri·ty
sal·u·tary
salve
sal·via
sam·ple
san·a·to·ri·um
san·da·rac
san·gui·fi·ca·tion
san·gui·nar·ia
san·guine
san·guin·e·ous
san·guin·o·lent
san·guis
sa·nies
san·i·tary
san·i·ta·tion
san·i·ty
sa·phe·na
sa·phe·nous
sap·id
sa·po
sa·po·na·ceous
sa·pon·i·fi·ca·tion
sa·po·nin
sap·phism
sa·pre·mia
sa·pre·mic
sap·ro·gen·ic

sar·a·pus
sar·ci·tis
sar·co·blast
sar·co·cele
sar·coid·osis
sar·co·lem·ma
sar·co·ma
sar·co·ma·to·sis
sar·co·ma·tous
sar·co·mere
sar·co·plasm
sar·cop·tes
sar·cous
sar·sa·pa·ril·la
sas·sa·fras
sat·el·lite
sat·el·lit·osis
sa·ti·ety
sat·u·rat·ed
sat·u·ra·tion
sat·ur·nine
sat·urn·ism
sa·ty·ri·a·sis
sau·cer·ize
sau·ri·a·sis
sau·sar·ism
scabbed
scab·i·cide
sca·bies
sca·bi·et·ic
sca·bi·ous
sca·bri·ti·es
sca·brous
sca·la
sca·lene
sca·le·nus

scal·ing
scalp
scal·pel
scaly
scan·sor·i·us
sca·pha
scaph·o·ceph·a·ly
scaph·oid
scap·u·la
scarf·skin
scar·i·fi·ca·tion
scar·la·ti·na
scar·la·ti·ni·form
scar·la·ti·noid
scarlet fe·ver
scav·en·ger
scav·eng·ing
scent
sche·ma
sche·mat·ic
schis·to·cyte
schis·to·so·mi·a·sis
schi·zog·o·ny
schiz·oid
schizo·phre·nia
schizo·phre·nic
schizo·thy·mic
schiz·o·thy·mous
schiz·o·trich·ia
sci·age
sci·at·ic
sci·at·i·ca
sci·e·ro·pia
scir·rhoid
scir·rhous adj.
scir·rhus n.

84

scis·sion
scis·sors
scis·su·ra
scis·sure
scle·ra
scle·rec·ta·sia
scle·rec·to·my
scle·re·ma
scle·ri·tis
scle·ro·blas·tema *or*
  scle·ro·blas·tem
scle·ro·blas·tem·ic
scle·rog·e·nous
scle·roid
scle·ro·ma
scle·rom·e·ter
scle·rose
scle·ro·sis
scle·ros·to·my
scle·ro·ther·a·py
scle·ro·thrix
scle·rot·ic
scle·ro·tium
scle·ro·tome
scle·rot·o·my
scle·rous
scob·i·nate
sco·le·coid
sco·lex
sco·li·o·lor·do·sis
sco·li·o·sis
sco·par·i·us
sco·po·la
sco·pol·amine
sco·po·phil·ia *or*
  scop·to·phil·ia

scor·a·cra·tia
scor·di·ne·ma
scot·o·din·ia
sco·to·ma
sco·tom·a·tous
sco·tom·e·ter
sco·to·pia
sco·to·pic
scro·bic·u·late
scro·bic·u·lus
scrof·u·la
scrof·u·lo·der·ma
scrof·u·lous
scro·tal
scro·tec·to·my
scro·tum
scru·pu·los·i·ty
scurf
scur·vy
scu·tate
scu·tu·lum
scu·tum
scy·phi·form
scy·ti·tis
sea·sick·ness
se·ba·ceous
se·ba·cic
se·bip·a·rous
seb·o·lith
se·bor·rhea
se·bor·rhe·ic
se·bum
se·cern·ment
se·clu·sion
sec·o·bar·bi·tal
sec·odont

sec·ond·ary
se·cre·ta
se·cre·ta·gogue
se·crete
se·cre·tin
se·cre·tin·ase
se·cre·tion
se·cre·to·ry
sec·tar·i·an
sec·tile
sec·tion
sec·to·ri·al
se·cun·di·grav·i·da
se·cun·dines
sec·un·dip·a·ra
sec·un·dip·a·rous
se·da·tion
sed·a·tive
sed·en·tary
sed·i·ment
sed·i·men·ta·ry
sed·i·men·ta·tion
seg·men·tal
seg·men·ta·tion
seg·re·ga·tion
seg·re·ga·tor
sei·es·the·sia
sei·zure
se·junc·tion
sel·a·pho·bia
se·lec·tion
se·le·ne
se·le·ni·ate
se·le·nic
sel·e·nif·er·ous
se·len·odont

sel·e·no·sis
self—ab·sorp·tion
self—fer·til·iza·tion
self—lim·it·ed
self—sus·pen·sion
sel·la *or* sel·lae
se·man·tics
se·men
semi·ca·nal
semi·car·ti·lag·i·nous
semi·co·ma
semi·co·ma·tose
semi·con·scious
semi·lu·nar
semi·lux·a·tion
semi·mem·bra·no·sus
semi·mem·bra·nous
sem·i·nal
sem·i·na·tion
sem·i·nif·er·ous
sem·i·no·ma
semi·nor·mal
semi·nu·ria
semi·pro·na·tion
semi·pto·sis
se·mis
semi·som·nous
semi·som·nus
semi·so·por
semi·spi·na·lis
semi·su·pi·na·tion
sem·i·ten·di·no·sus
sem·i·ten·di·nous

se·nec·ti·tude
sen·e·ga *or* sen·e·ca
se·nes·cence
se·nile
se·nil·ism
se·nil·i·ty
se·ni·um
se·no·pia
sen·sa·tion
sense
sen·si·bil·i·ty
sen·si·bi·liz·er
sen·si·ble
sen·si·tive
sen·si·tiv·i·ty
sen·so·ri·mo·tor
sen·so·ri·um
sen·so·ry
sen·su·al
sen·sus
sen·tient
sep·a·rate
sep·a·ra·tion n. (act of dividing; cf. *suppression, suppuration*)
sep·a·ra·tor
sep·sis
sep·tal
sep·tic
sep·ti·ce·mia
sep·ti·co·phle·bi·tis
sep·ti·grav·i·da
sep·tip·a·ra
sep·tom·e·ter

sep·to·tome
sep·tu·lum
sep·tum
sep·tup·let
sep·ul·ture
se·que·la
se·quence
se·quen·tial
se·ques·ter·ing
se·que·stra·tion
se·ques·trec·to·my
se·ques·trum
sere·noa
se·ries
ser·ine
se·ri·ous adj. (grave; cf. *serous*)
se·ro·cul·ture
se·ro·der·ma·to·sis
se·ro·di·ag·no·sis
se·ro·log·i·cal·ly
se·rol·o·gist
se·rol·o·gy
se·ro·mu·cous
se·ro·per·i·to·ne·um
se·ro·pu·ru·lent
se·ro·re·ac·tion
se·ro·re·sis·tance
se·ro·re·sis·tant
se·ro·sa
se·ro·se·rous
se·ro·si·tis
se·ro·ther·a·py
se·rous adj. (having nature of serum; cf. *serious*)

ser·pens
ser·pen·tar·ia
ser·pig·i·nous
ser·ra
ser·rate
ser·ra·tia
ser·ra·tion
ser·ra·tus
se·rum sing.
se·rums or se·ra pl.
ser·vo·mech·a·nism
ses·a·me
ses·a·moid·itis
ses·qui·ho·ra
ses·sile
se·ta
se·ton
se·vip·a·rous
se·vum
sex·ol·o·gy
sex·ti·grav·i·da
sex·tip·a·ra
sex·tu·plet
sex·u·al·i·ty
shad·ow
shank
shears
sheath n.
shed·ding
shel·tered
shield
shi·gel·la
shig·el·lo·sis
shin
shin·gles
shiv·er

shoul·der
shriv·eled or
    shriv·elled
shud·der
shunt
si·al·a·den
si·al·a·gogue
si·al·a·po·ria
si·al·ic
si·a·lo·a·er·oph·a·gy
si·a·log·e·nous
si·a·log·ra·phy
si·a·loid
si·al·o·lith
si·al·o·li·thi·a·sis
si·al·or·rhea
sib·i·lant
sib·i·la·tion
sib·i·lis·mus
sib·i·lus
sib·ling
sib·ship
sic·cant
sic·ca·tive
sic·cha·sia
sic·cus
sid·er·o·phile
sid·er·oph·i·lin
sid·er·o·sis
sid·er·ot·ic
sig·ma·tism
sig·moid·ec·to·my
sig·moid·itis
sig·moid·o·scope
sig·moid·o·scop·ic
sig·moid·os·to·my

sig·na pl.
sig·na·ture
sig·nif·i·cant
sig·num sing.
si·lent
sil·i·ca
sil·i·cate
sil·i·ca·to·sis
si·li·ceous or
    si·li·cious
si·lic·ic
si·li·ci·um
sil·i·con
sil·i·co·sis
sil·ver
sim·ple
sim·u·la·tion
si·na·pis
sin·a·pism
sin·ci·put
sin·ew
sin·gul·tus
sin·is·ter
si·ni·stra
sin·is·trad
sin·is·tral·i·ty
sin·is·tra·tion
sin·is·trau·ral
sin·is·tro·car·di·al
sin·is·tro·cer·e·bral
sin·is·troc·u·lar
sin·is·tro·gy·ra·tion
sin·is·tro·gy·ric
sin·is·tro·man·u·al
sin·is·trop·e·dal
sin·is·tror·sal·ly

sin·is·trorse
sin·is·tro·sis
sin·is·tro·tor·tion
si·nis·trous
si·no·atri·al
si·no·bron·chi·tis
si·nom·e·nine
sin·u·ous
si·nus·itis
si·nus·oid
si·nus·oi·dal·ly
si·nus·ot·o·my
si·phon·age
si·phon·ap·tera
si·ri·a·sis
si·tol·o·gy
si·to·ma·nia
si·to·pho·bia
si·to·ther·a·py
si·tus
skat·ole
ske·lal·gia
skel·e·tal
skel·e·ti·za·tion
skel·e·ton
ske·nei·tis
skene·o·scope
skew
skia·gram
ski·ag·ra·phy
ski·am·e·try
skia·scope
ski·as·co·py
skull·cap
slake
slap·ping

sla·ver v.
slav·er n.
sleep·less·ness
slic·er
sling
slough
sludge
slum·ber
small·pox
smear
smeg·ma
smeg·mat·ic
smudg·ing
sneeze
sniff·ing
snif·fling
snore
snow blind·ness
so·cial
so·ci·ety
so·cio·log·ic
so·ci·ol·o·gy
so·cio·med·i·cal
so·ci·o·path·ic
sock·et
so·cor·dia
so·da·mide
so·di·um
sod·omy
soft·en·ing
so·la·na·ce·ae
so·la·na·ceous
so·la·na·nine or so-
la·nin
so·la·num
so·lar·iza·tion

so·lar plex·us
so·las·o·dine
so·las·o·nine
so·la·tion
so·la·ti·um
sole (of foot)
so·lei pl.
sole·plate
so·le·us sing.
so·lid·i·fi·ca·tion
so·lid·i·fy
so·lip·sism
sol·i·tary
sol·u·bil·i·ty
sol·u·bi·lize
sol·u·ble
solu·nar
so·lute
so·lu·tion
sol·vate
sol·va·tion
sol·vent
so·ma
so·mat·es·the·sia
so·mat·i·cal·ly
so·ma·tist
so·ma·ti·za·tion
so·ma·to·chrome
so·ma·to·gen·ic
so·ma·tog·e·ny
so·ma·tol·o·gy
so·ma·tome
so·ma·to·meg·a·ly
so·ma·to·met·ric
so·ma·tom·e·try
so·ma·to·path·ic

so·ma·to·plasm
so·ma·to·pleur·al
so·ma·to·pleure
so·ma·to·psy·chic
so·ma·to·to·nia
so·ma·to·top·ic
so·ma·tot·ro·pin
so·ma·to·type
som·es·the·sia
som·es·thet·ic
so·mite
som·nam·bu·lism
som·nam·bu·list
som·nam·bu·lis·tic
som·ni·fa·cient
som·nif·er·ous
som·nif·ic
som·nif·u·gous
som·nil·o·quy
om·nip·a·thy
som·no·lence
som·no·lent
om·no·len·tia
om·no·les·cent
om·no·lism
som·nus
one
o·no·chem·is·try
o·pho·ra
oph·o·rine
o·por
o·po·rif·er·ous
o·po·rif·ic
o·po·rose
or·bic
or·bi·tan

sor·bit·ic
sor·bose
sor·des
sore
so·ro·ri·a·tion
spall·ation
spar·a·drap
spar·ga·num
spar·go·sis
spar·te·ine
spasm
spas·mat·ic
spas·mat·i·cal
spas·mod·ic
spas·mod·i·cal·ly
spas·mo·gen·ic
spas·mol·y·sis
spas·mo·lyt·ic
spas·mo·phil·ia
spas·mo·phil·ic
spas·mus
spas·tic
spas·ti·cal·ly
spas·tic·i·ty
spa·tial
spa·ti·um
spat·u·la
spat·u·late
spay
spear·mint
spe·cial·ist
spe·cial·iza·tion
spe·cies
spe·cif·ic
spe·cif·i·cal·ly
spec·i·fi·ca·tion

spec·i·fic·i·ty
spec·i·fy
spec·i·men
spec·ta·cles
spec·tro·gram
spec·tro·graph
spec·trom·e·ter
spec·trom·e·try
spec·tro·scope
spec·tro·scop·ic
spec·tros·co·py
spec·trum
spec·u·lum
sperm
sper·mat·ic
sper·mat·i·cal·ly
sper·ma·tid
sper·ma·to·cele
sper·ma·to·cide
sper·ma·to·cyst
sper·ma·to·cys·tic
sper·ma·to·cyte
sper·ma·to·gen·ic
sper·ma·tog·e·nous
sper·ma·to·go·ni·um
sper·ma·toid
sper·ma·tol·y·sis
sper·ma·to·lyt·ic
sper·ma·top·a·thy
sper·ma·to·phore
sper·ma·tor·rhea
sper·ma·tox·in
sper·ma·to·zo·id
sper·ma·to·zo·on
sper·ma·tu·ria
sper·mec·to·my

sper·mi·a·tion
sper·mi·cide
sperm·ine
sper·mo·lith
sphac·e·late
sphac·e·lism
sphac·e·lo·der·ma
sphac·e·lous
sphac·e·lus
spha·gi·as·mus
spha·gi·tis
sphe·ni·on
sphe·no·ceph·a·ly
sphe·noid
sphe·noi·dal
sphe·noid·itis
sphe·no·pa·ri·e·tal
sphe·no·sis
sphere
spher·ic
spher·i·cal
sphero·cyte
sphero·cyt·ic
sphero·cy·to·sis
spher·oid
sphe·roi·dal
sphe·rom·e·ter
spher·ule
sphinc·ter
sphinc·ter·al·gia
sphinc·ter·ot·o·my
sphin·go·sine
sphyg·mic·al
sphyg·mo·bo·lom-
   e·ter
sphyg·mod·ic

sphyg·mo·graph·ic
sphyg·mog·ra·phy
sphyg·moid
sphyg·mo·ma·nom-
   e·ter
sphyg·mo·pal·pa-
   tion
sphyg·mo·sys·to·le
sphyg·mo·to·nom-
   e·ter
sphyg·mous
sphyg·mus
spi·ca
spic·u·la
spi·der
spike
spik·i·ly
spi·lus
spi·na   bi·fi·da
spi·nal
spi·na·lis
spin·dle
spin·dling
spin·dly
spine
spi·no·tec·tal
spi·nous
spin·thari·scope
spin·ther·ism
spi·nu·lo·sa
spi·raled   or
   spi·ralled
spi·ral·ing   or
   spi·ral·ling
spi·ril·lo·sis
spi·ril·lum

spir·it
spi·ro·chae·ta
spi·ro·chae·ta·ce·ae
spi·ro·chae·ta·les
spi·ro·chete   or
   spi·ro·chaete
spi·ro·chet·emia
spi·ro·che·ti·cide
spi·ro·chet·osis
spi·ro·gram
spi·rom·e·ter
spi·ro·met·ric
spi·rom·e·try
spis·si·tude
spiz·en·stoss
splanch·na
splanch·nec·to·pia
splanch·nem-
   phrax·is
splanch·nes·the·sia
splanch·neu·rys·ma
splanch·nic
splanch·ni·cec·to·m
splanch·ni·cot·o·my
splanch·no·coel   or
   splanch·no·coele
splanch·no·meg·a·ly
splanch·nop·a·thy
splanch·no·pleu·ral
splanch·no·pleure
splanch·nop·to·sis
splanch·nos·co·py
splanch·not·o·my
splanch·no·tribe
spleen
sple·nal·gia

90

ple·nec·to·mize
ple·nec·to·my
ple·net·ic
ple·nic
plen·i·form
ple·ni·tis
ple·ni·us
pleni·za·tion
pleno·cele
pleno·cyte
pleno·dyn·ia
pleno·gen·ic
ple·noid
ple·no·meg·a·ly
ple·nop·a·thy
pleno·pexy
ple·nor·rha·phy
ple·not·o·my
plice
plint *or* splent
plint·age
plin·ter
plint·ing
plit·ting
poke·shave
pon·dy·lal·gia
pon·dy·lit·ic
pon·dy·li·tis
pon·dy·lo·lis·
  the·sis
pon·dyl·op·a·thy
pon·dy·lo·sis
pon·dy·lo·syn·de·
  sis
pon·dy·lot·o·my
ponge

spon·gi·form
spon·gi·o·blas·to·
  ma
spon·gi·o·cyte
spon·gi·ose
spon·gi·o·sis
spon·gi·ous
spongy
spon·ta·ne·ous
spo·rad·ic
spo·rad·i·cal·ly
spo·ran·gi·um
spore
spo·ri·ci·dal
spo·ro·cyst
spo·ro·cyte
spo·ro·gen·e·sis
spo·rog·e·nous
spo·rog·o·ny
spo·ro·tri·cho·sis
spo·rot·ri·chum
spo·ro·zoa
spo·ro·zo·an
spo·ro·zo·ite
spo·ro·zo·on
spor·u·late
spot·ting
sprain
spread·ing
sprue
spur
spu·tum
squa·ma
squame
squa·mo—oc·cip·i·
  tal

squa·mo·sa
squa·mous
squint
stabbed
stab·bing
sta·bi·liz·er
sta·ble
stac·ca·to
stach·y·ose
sta·di·um
stag·na·tion
stain
stam·i·na
stam·mer·ing
stan·dard·iza·tion
stand·still
stan·nate
stan·nic
sta·pe·des (sing.:
  stapes)
sta·pe·di·al
sta·pe·dio·ves·
  tib·u·lar
sta·pe·di·us
sta·pes (pl.: *stapes* or
  stapedes)
staph·y·le·de·ma
staph·y·le·us
staph·y·line
sta·phyl·i·on
staph·y·lo·coc·cal
staph·y·lo·coc·ce·
  mia
staph·y·lo·coc·cic
staph·y·lo·coc·cus
staph·y·lo·ma

staph·y·lo·mat·ic
staph·y·lom·atous
staph·y·lot·o·my
star·blind
starch·i·ness
starchy
star·va·tion
starv·ing
sta·sis (stoppage of
   flow; cf. *staxis*)
stat·ics
stat·im
sta·tion
sta·tis·ti·cal
sta·tis·tics
stat·o·ki·net·ic
stat·ure
sta·tus quo
stau·ri·on
stax·is (hemorrhage;
   cf. *stasis*)
stea·rate
stea·ric
stear·i·form
stea·rin
stea·ryl
ste·a·tin
ste·a·ti·tis
ste·a·tog·e·nous
ste·atol·y·sis
ste·a·to·ma
ste·ato·py·gia
ste·ato·pyg·ic
ste·ato·py·gous
ste·ator·rhea
ste·a·to·sis

steg·no·sis
steg·not·ic
stego·my·ia
stel·late·ly
stel·lec·to·my
steni·on
steno·ceph·a·ly
steno·chas·mus
steno·cho·ria
steno·co·ri·a·sis
steno·dont
steno·mer·ic
steno·pe·ic
ste·nosed
ste·no·sis
steno·sto·mia
ste·nos·to·my
steno·ther·mal
steno·tho·rax
stent
sten·to·roph·o-
   nous
ste·pha·ni·on
step·page gait
ster·co·bi·lin
ster·co·bi·lin·o·gen
ster·co·ra·ceous
ster·co·rary
ster·co·ro·ma
ster·cus
stere
ste·reo·blas·tu·la
ste·re·og·no·sis
ste·re·og·nos·tic
ste·reo·gram
ste·re·og·ra·phy

ste·reo·iso·mer
ste·re·op·sis
ste·re·op·ter
ste·reo·scope
ste·reo·scop·ic
ste·re·os·co·py
ste·reo·tax·ia
ste·reo·tax·is
ste·re·ot·ro·pism
ste·reo·ty·py
ster·ic hin·drance
ster·id
ster·ile
ste·ril·i·ty
ster·il·iza·tion
ster·il·ize
ster·il·iz·er
ster·na·lis
ster·no·cla·vic·u·la
ster·no·hy·oid
ster·no·thy·roid
ster·not·o·my
ster·num
ster·nu·ta·tion
ster·nu·ta·tor
ste·roid
ste·rol
ster·tor
ster·to·rous
stetho·scope
stetho·scop·ic
ste·tho·sco·py
sthe·nia
sthen·ic
stib·i·al·ism
stic·ta

stic·tac·ne
sti·fle
stig·ma·tism
stig·ma·ti·za·tion
stig·ma·tose
still·birth
still·born
stim·u·lant
stim·u·late
stim·u·la·tion
stim·u·li pl.
stim·u·lus sing.
stip·pling
stitch
stock·i·nette or
    stock·i·net
stoi·chi·om·e·try
sto·ma
stom·ach
sto·mach·ic
sto·mat·ic
sto·ma·ti·tis
stoma·to·gas·tric
sto·ma·tol·o·gy
sto·ma·to·mia
sto·mat·o·my
sto·ma·to·sis
sto·mo·dae·um or
    sto·mo·de·um
stool
stop·page
sto·rax
stra·bis·mal
stra·bis·mic
stra·bis·mus
strag·u·lum

strain
strait·jack·et or
    straight·jack·et
stra·mo·ni·um
stran·gle
stran·gu·la·tion
stran·gu·ry
stra·ta pl.
strat·i·fi·ca·tion
strat·i·fied
stra·tig·ra·phy
strato·sphere
stra·tum sing.
straw·ber·ry
    mark
strep·i·tus
strep·to·an·gi·na
strep·to·ba·cil·lus
strep·to·coc·cal
strep·to·coc·cic
strep·to·coc·cus
strep·to·dor·nase
strep·to·ki·nase
strep·to·ly·sin
strep·to·my·ces
strep·to·my·cin
strep·to·thri·cin
stretch·er
stria
stri·at·ed
stri·a·tion
stri·a·tum
strick·en
stric·ture
stri·dor
strid·u·lous

strin·gent
strip·ping
strob·ic
stro·bi·la
stro·bi·la·tion
stro·bile
strob·i·loid
stro·bi·lus
stro·ma
stro·mal
stro·ma·tal
stro·mat·ic
stro·ma·tin
stro·muhr
stron·tium
stro·phan·thin
stro·phan·thus
stroph·o·ceph·a·ly
stroph·u·lus
struc·tur·al
struc·ture
stru·ma
stru·mi·form
stru·mi·priv·al
stru·mi·pri·vous
stru·mi·tis
stru·mous
strych·nine
strych·nin·iza·tion
stub·bi·ness
stub·by
stun
stunt·ing
stupe
stu·pe·fa·cient
stu·pe·fac·tion

stu·pe·fy·ing
stu·por
stut·ter·ing
sty·let
sty·lo·glos·sus
sty·lus
styp·tic
sub·ab·dom·i·nal
sub·acute
sub·al·i·men·ta·tion
sub·api·cal
sub·arach·noid
sub·au·ric·u·lar
sub·cla·vi·an
sub·cla·vi·us
sub·clin·i·cal
sub·con·scious
sub·con·tin·u·ous
sub·cor·a·coid
sub·cor·ti·cal
sub·cos·tal
sub·crep·i·tant
sub·crep·i·ta·tion
sub·cul·ture
sub·cu·ta·ne·ous
sub·cu·tic·u·lar
sub·cu·tis
sub·di·vid·ed
sub·duct
sub·duc·tion
sub·du·ral
sub·glos·si·tis
su·bic·u·lum
sub·in·ci·sion
sub·in·fec·tion

sub·in·vo·lu·tion
sub·ja·cent
sub·jec·tive
sub·la·tion
sub·le·thal
sub·li·mate
sub·li·ma·tion
sub·li·mi·nal
sub·lin·gual
sub·max·il·lary
sub·men·tal
sub·mu·co·sa
sub·mu·cous
sub·nar·cot·ic
sub·nor·mal
sub·nor·mal·i·ty
sub·nu·cle·us
sub·nu·tri·tion
sub·oc·cip·i·tal
sub·or·di·na·tion
sub·peri·os·te·al
sub·pla·cen·ta
sub·plan·ti·grade
sub·pu·bic
sub·scap·u·lar
sub·scap·u·lar·is
sub·scrip·tion
sub·se·rous
sub·si·dence
sub·sis·tence
sub·spi·nous
sub·stance
sub·stan·tia
sub·ster·nal
sub·sti·tu·tion
sub·strate

sub·sul·to·ry
sub·sul·tus
sub·ten·to·ri·al
sub·thal·a·mus
sub·u·ber·es
sub·un·gual
sub·un·gui·al
suc·ce·da·ne·ous
suc·cor·rhea *or*
   suc·cor·rhoea
suc·cu·bus
suc·cu·lent
suc·cur·sal
suc·cus·sion
suck·ing
suck·ling
su·crose
suc·tion
suc·to·ri·al
su·da·men
su·da·tion
su·da·to·ria pl.
su·da·to·ri·um sing.
su·dor
su·do·re·sis
su·do·rif·er·ous
su·do·rif·ic
su·do·rip·a·rous
suf·fo·cate
suf·fo·ca·tion
suf·fu·sion
sug·ar
sug·gest·ibil·i·ty
sug·gest·ible
sug·ges·tion
sug·gil·la·tion

sui·ci·dal
sui·cide
su·int
sul·cus
sul·fa
sul·fa·di·a·zine
sul·fa·nil·amide
sul·fate
sul·fa·thi·a·zole
sul·fide or sul·phide
sul·fon·amide
sul·fur or sul·phur
sul·fu·ric or sul·phu·ric
sul·fu·rous or sul·phu·rous
sul·lage
sul·len
su·mac or su·mach
sum·ma·tion
sun·burned
sun·lamp
sun·stroke
su·per·ab·duc·tion
su·per·ac·id
su·per·acid·i·ty
su·per·ac·tiv·i·ty
su·per·acute
su·per·al·i·men·ta·tion
su·per·cil·i·ary
su·per·cil·i·um
su·per·duct
su·per·ego
su·per·ex·ten·tion

su·per·fe·cun·da·tion
su·per·fe·cun·di·ty
su·per·fe·ta·tion
su·per·fi·cial
su·per·fi·ci·al·i·ty
su·per·fi·cies
su·per·im·preg·na·tion
su·per·in·duce
su·per·in·fec·tion
su·pe·ri·or·i·ty
su·per·lac·ta·tion
su·per·nate
su·per·nu·mer·ary
su·per·nu·tri·tion
su·per·scrip·tion
su·per·se·cre·tion
su·per·sen·si·tive
su·per·ten·sion
su·per·ven·tion
su·per·vi·sor
su·pi·na·tion
su·pi·na·tor
su·pine
sup·pe·da·ne·ous
sup·pe·da·ne·um
sup·ple·men·tal
sup·ple·men·ta·ry
sup·ple·men·ta·tion
sup·port·er
sup·pos·i·to·ry
sup·pres·sion (sudden stoppage; cf. *separation, suppuration*)

sup·pu·rant
sup·pu·rate
sup·pu·ra·tion (formation of pus; cf. *separation, suppression*)
sup·pu·ra·tive
su·pra·cho·roid
su·pra·cla·vic·u·lar
su·pra·glot·tic
su·pra·hy·oid
su·pra·li·mi·nal
su·pra·mas·toid
su·pra·oc·clu·sion
su·pra·or·bit·al
su·pra·pu·bic
su·pra·re·nal
su·pra·re·nal·ec·to·my
su·pra·ren·a·lin
su·pra·scap·u·la
su·pra·scap·u·lar
su·pra·sel·lar
su·pra·spi·na·tus
su·pra·spi·nous
su·pra·ster·nal
su·pra·ton·sil·lar
su·pra·troch·le·ar
su·pra·ver·gence
su·pra·vi·tal
su·ra
sur·al·i·men·ta·tion
sur·a·min
surd·i·ty
sur·ex·ci·ta·tion
sur·face

sur·geon
sur·gery
sur·gi·cal
sur·ra
sur·ro·gate
sur·sum·duc·tion
sur·sum·ver·gence
sur·sum·ver·sion
sur·vi·vor·ship
sus·cep·ti·bil·i·ty
sus·cep·ti·ble
sus·cep·tive
sus·cep·tiv·i·ty
sus·ci·tate
sus·pend·ed
sus·pen·sion
sus·pen·soid
sus·pen·so·ri·um
sus·pen·so·ry
sus·pi·ra·tion
sus·ten·tac·u·lum
su·sur·ra·tion
su·sur·rous adj.
su·sur·rus n.
su·tu·ra
su·tur·al
su·ture
swab stick
swal·low·ing
sweat·ing
swell·ing
sy·co·ma
sy·co·sis (inflamma-
    tion of hair follicles;
    cf: *psychosis*)
sym·bi·o·sis

sym·bi·ot·ic
sym·bleph·a·ron
sym·met·ric
sym·met·ri·cal
sym·me·try
sym·pa·thec·to·my
sym·pa·thet·ic
sym·pa·thet·i·co-
    blas·to·ma
sym·pa·thin
sym·pa·thism
sym·pa·thiz·er
sym·pa·tho·mi·met-
    ic
sym·pa·thy
sym·pha·lan·gism
sym·phy·sis
symp·tom·at·ic
symp·tom·atol·o·gy
symp·to·sis
sym·pus
syn·ac·to·sis
syn·al·gia
syn·an·che
syn·an·the·ma
syn·apse
syn·ar·thro·phy·sis
syn·ar·thro·sis
syn·ceph·a·lus
syn·chon·dro·sis
syn·chon·drot·o·my
syn·chro·nism
syn·chy·sis
syn·clo·nus
syn·co·pal
syn·co·pe

syn·dac·tyl or
    syn·dac·tyle
syn·dac·ty·ly
syn·de·sis
syn·des·mi·tis
syn·des·mo·sis
syn·des·mot·ic
syn·des·mot·o·my
syn·drome
syn·dro·mic
syn·ech·ia
syn·er·e·sis
syn·er·get·ic
syn·er·gic
syn·er·gism
syn·er·gist
syn·er·gis·tic
syn·er·gy
syn·es·the·sia
syn·es·thet·ic
syn·ga·my
syn·ge·ne·sious
syn·gig·no·scism
syn·hi·dro·sis
syn·i·ze·sis
syn·kary·on
syn·ki·ne·sia
syn·oph·rys
syn·os·tosed
syn·os·to·sis
syn·ovi·o·ma
syn·o·vi·tis
syn·ta·sis
syn·the·sis
syn·thet·ic
syn·ton·ic

syn·tro·phus
syph·i·lid
syph·i·lis
syph·i·lit·ic
syph·i·lo·derm *or*
  syph·i·lo·der·ma
syph·i·loid
syph·i·lo·ma
syph·i·lo·pho·bia
syph·i·lo·phy·ma
syph·i·lo·ther·a·py
Sy·rette
sy·rig·mus
syr·ing·ad·e·no·sus
sy·ringe·ful
syr·in·go·ma
syr·up
sys·sar·co·sis
sys·tal·tic
sys·tem·ic
sys·tem·i·cal·ly
sys·to·le
sys·tol·ic
sys·trem·ma
syz·y·gy

T

tab·a·co·sis
ta·bel·la

ta·bes dor·sa·lis
ta·bet·ic
ta·bet·i·form
ta·ble·spoon
tab·let
tab·u·lar
tache *or* tach
ta·chet·ic
ta·chis·to·scope
ta·chis·to·scop·ic
tachy·aux·e·sis
tachy·car·dia (rapid
  heart action; cf.
  bradycardia)
tachy·car·di·ac
tachy·graph
ta·chyg·ra·phy
tachy·lo·gia
tachy·pha·gia
tachy·pnea
tachy·rhyth·mia
ta·chys·ter·ol
tachy·sys·to·le
tac·tile
tac·toid
tae·di·um vi·tae
tae·nia
tae·nia·cide
tae·nia·fuge
tae·ni·a·sis
tae·ni·form
tae·ni·oid
tag·ma
taint
ta·lal·gia
talc

tal·cum
tali·pes
tal·i·pom·a·nus
tal·low
ta·lus
tam·pon
tam·pon·ade
tan·nic
tan·sy
tan·ta·lum
tan·trum
ta·pe·tum
tape·worm
taph·e·pho·bia
tap·i·o·ca
tap·ping
ta·ran·tu·la
ta·rax·is
tar·dive
tare
tar·get
tar·si·tis
tar·sor·rha·phy
tar·sus
tar·tar
tar·tar·e·ous
tar·tar·ic
tar·tra·zine
tat·too·ing
tau·rine
tau·to·me·ni·al
tau·tom·er·al
tax·is
tax·o·nom·ic
tax·on·o·my
tears

tease
tea·spoon
teat
tech·ne·tium
tech·nic
tech·nique
tec·ti·form
tec·tum
te·dious·ness
teeth·ing
teg·men
teg·men·tum *or*
  teg·u·men·tum
te·la
tel·an·gi·ec·ta·sis
tel·an·gi·i·tis
te·leg·o·ny
tele·ki·ne·sis
te·le·o·log·i·cal
te·le·ol·o·gy
te·lep·a·thist
te·lep·a·thy
tel·es·the·sia
tele·ther·a·py
tel·lu·ri·um
te·lo·phase
tem·per·a·ment
tem·per·ance
tem·per·ate
tem·per·a·ture
tem·ple
tem·po·ral
tem·po·rary
tem·po·ri·za·tion
te·na·cious
te·nac·i·ty

te·nac·u·lum
ten·der·ness
ten·di·nous
ten·do
ten·don
ten·don·ous
ten·do·vag·i·ni·tis
te·nec·to·my
te·nes·mus
ten·i·o·la
ten·nis el·bow
ten·o·de·sis
ten·on·i·tis
ten·o·phyte
ten·or·rha·phy
ten·os·to·sis
te·no·syn·o·vi·tis
ten·o·tome
te·not·o·mize
te·not·o·my
tense·ness
ten·sion
ten·si·ty
ten·sive
ten·sor
ten·sure
ten·ta·tive
ten·tig·i·nous
ten·ti·go
ten·to·ri·al
ten·to·ri·um
ten·u·ate
te·nu·ity
ten·u·ous·ly
ter·a·tism
ter·a·to·ma

ter·a·to·ma·tous
ter·a·to·sis
te·re
te·res
ter·mi·nal
ter·mi·nate
ter·mi·na·tion
ter·mi·nol·o·gy
ter·na·ry
ter·pene
ter·ra
Ter·ra·my·cin
ter·tian
ter·ti·ary
ter·tip·a·ra
tes·ta·ceous
tes·tes pl.
tes·ti·cle
tes·tic·u·lar
tes·tis sing.
tes·tos·ter·one
tet·a·nal
te·tan·ic
te·tan·i·form
tet·a·nig·e·nous
tet·a·nism
tet·a·ni·za·tion
tet·a·node
tet·a·nus
tet·a·ny
te·tar·to·cone
te·tar·to·co·nid
tet·ra·caine
tet·rad
tet·ra·dac·tyl
tet·ter

tex·is
tex·tur·al
tex·ture
tex·tus
thal·a·mus
thal·as·se·mia
tha·mu·ria
than·a·toid
than·a·tos
the·ca
the·cal
the·ci·tis
the·co·dont
the·co·steg·no·sis
the·ine
the·ism
the·lal·gia
the·las·is
the·ler·e·thism
the·li·on
the·li·tis
the·li·um
the·nar
theo·bro·mine
theo·ma·nia
theo·pho·bia
theo·phyl·line
the·o·ret·i·cal
the·o·ry
ther·a·peu·sis
ther·a·peu·ti·cal·ly
ther·a·peu·tics
ther·a·peu·tist
the·ra·pia
ther·a·pist
ther·a·py

the·ri·a·ca
the·ri·od·ic
the·ri·o·ma
ther·mal
ther·mal·ge·sia
therm·es·the·sia
ther·mic
ther·mo·cau·tery
ther·mo·chem·is·try
ther·mo·du·ric
ther·mo·gen·ic
ther·mog·e·nous
ther·mol·y·sis
ther·mo·lyt·ic
ther·mom·e·ter
ther·mo·met·ric
ther·moph·a·gy
ther·mo·phile (organ-
    ism)
ther·mo·phil·ic
ther·mo·phore
ther·mo·pile (ap-
    paratus)
ther·mo·ple·gia
ther·mo·pol·yp·nea
ther·mo·stat·i·
    cal·ly
ther·mo·tax·is
ther·mo·ther·a·py
the·sis
thi·ami·nase
thi·a·mine
thi·a·zole
thigh
thig·mes·the·sia
thi·mer·o·sal

thio·chrome
thio·glyc·er·ol
thi·one·ine
thi·on·ic
thio·pen·tone
thio·phene
thi·o·phil·ic
thio·urea
thixo·trop·ic
thix·ot·ro·py
tho·ra·cec·to·my
tho·ra·cen·te·sis
tho·rac·ic
tho·rac·i·co·lum·bar
    or tho·ra·co·
    lum·bar
tho·ra·co·dyn·ia
tho·ra·cop·a·gus
tho·ra·co·plas·ty
tho·ra·co·scope
tho·ra·co·scop·ic
tho·ra·cos·to·my
tho·ra·cot·o·my
tho·rax
tho·ri·um
thread·ed
threp·sol·o·gy
thresh·old
thrill
throat
throb
throe
throm·bas·the·nia
throm·bec·to·my
throm·bin
throm·bo·an·gi·i·tis

99

throm·bo·ar·te·ri·tis
throm·bo·blast
throm·boc·la·sis
throm·bo·cyte
throm·bo·cyt·ic
throm·bo·cy·to·pe·nia
throm·bo·cy·to·poi·e·sis
throm·bo·cy·to·sis
throm·bo·em·bol·ic
throm·bo·gen·ic
throm·bo·ki·nase
throm·bo·pe·nia
throm·bo·phle·bi·tis
throm·bo·plas·tic
throm·bosed
throm·bo·sis
throm·bot·ic
throm·bus
throt·tle
throw back v.
throw·back n.
thrush
thumb
thyme
thy·mec·to·my
thym·ic (of thyme)
thy·mic (of thymus)
thy·mi·on
thy·mi·tis
thy·mo·cyte
thy·mol
thy·mo·ma

thy·mo·no·ic
thy·mop·a·thy
thy·mus
thy·ro·ad·e·ni·tis
thy·ro·cele
thy·rog·e·nous
thy·ro·glob·u·lin
thy·ro·glos·sal
thy·roid·ec·to·my
thy·roid·i·tis
thy·roid·iza·tion
thy·roid·ot·o·my
thy·ro·pri·val
thy·ro·sis
thy·rot·o·my
thy·ro·tox·ic
thy·ro·tox·i·co·sis
thy·rox·ine or thy·rox·in
tib·ia
tib·i·al
tib·i·alis
tib·io·fib·u·lar
tic (spasmodic motion)
tick (parasite)
tick·le
tick·ling
tic·tol·o·gy
tim·bre
tim·o·thy
tinc·to·ri·al
tinc·ture
tine
tin·ea
tin·gle
tin·ni·tus

tint·om·e·ter
tint·o·met·ric
tint·om·e·try
ti·queur
tis·sue
ti·ta·ni·um
ti·ter or ti·tre
tit·il·la·tion
ti·tra·tion
tit·u·ba·tion
to·bac·co
to·coph·er·ol
to·cus
to·kol·o·gy
to·kom·e·try
to·ko·pho·bia
tol·er·ance
tol·er·ant
tol·er·a·tion
to·lu·ic
tol·u·yl·ene
tom·a·tine
to·men·tum
to·mo·to·cia
ton·al
tongue—tied
ton·ic
to·nic·i·ty
ton·i·tro·pho·bia
to·nom·e·ter
ton·sil
ton·sil·lar
ton·sil·lec·tome
ton·sil·lec·to·my
ton·sil·lit·ic
ton·sil·li·tis

ton·sil·lo·tome
ton·sil·lot·o·my
ton·sure
to·nus
tooth·ache
toothed
toothpaste
tooth pow·der
to·pal·gia
to·pec·to·my
top·es·the·sia
to·pha·ceous
to·phus
top·i·cal
to·pol·o·gy
top·o·nar·co·sis
top·o·neu·ro·sis
tor·mi·na
tor·mi·nal
tor·mi·nous
tor·pid·i·ty
tor·por
torque
tor·sion
tor·sive
tor·so
tor·soc·clu·sion
tor·ti·col·lar
tor·ti·col·lis
tor·tu·ous (winding)
tor·u·lus
to·rus
to·ta·quine
to·tip·o·tence
to·ti·po·tent
tour·ni·quet

tox·emia
tox·emic
tox·ic
tox·i·cant
tox·ic·i·ty
tox·i·co·den·drol
tox·i·co·den·dron
tox·i·co·der·ma
tox·i·co·gen·ic
tox·i·coid
tox·i·co·log·ic
tox·i·col·o·gist
tox·i·co·sis
tox·if·er·ous
tox·ig·e·nous
tox·in
toxi·ta·bel·lae
tox·oid
tox·on·o·sis
tox·oph·o·rous
tox·o·plas·ma
toxo·plas·mo·sis
tra·chea
tra·che·al
tra·che·al·gia
tra·che·i·tis
tra·che·li·um
tra·che·lo·mas·toid
tra·che·lor·rha·phy
tra·che·lot·o·my
tra·che·o·cele
tra·che·os·to·my
tra·che·ot·o·mize
tra·che·ot·o·my
tra·cho·ma
tra·cho·ma·tous

tra·chy·chro·mat·ic
tra·chy·pho·nia
tract
trac·tion
trac·tot·o·my
trac·tus
trade·mark
trag·a·canth
tra·gi pl.
tra·gus sing.
trait
trance
trans·an·i·ma·tion
trans·au·di·ent
trans·ca·lent
trans·con·dy·lar
trans·duc·tion
tran·sec·tion
trans·fer·ence
trans·fix·ion
trans·for·ma·tion
trans·form·er
trans·fuse
trans·fu·sion·ist
tran·sient
trans·il·i·ac
trans·il·lu·mi·na·tion
tran·sis·tor
tran·si·tion·al
trans·lu·cent
trans·lu·cid
trans·mi·gra·tion
trans·mis·si·bil·i·ty
trans·mis·sion

trans·mit·tance
trans·mu·ta·tion
trans·mute
trans·o·nance
trans·par·ent
tran·spir·able
tran·spi·ra·tion
trans·plant
trans·plan·ta·tion
trans·pose
trans·po·si·tion
tran·sub·stan·ti·a-
  tion
tran·sud·ate
tran·su·da·tion
tran·sude
trans·ure·thral
trans·vag·i·nal
trans·ver·sa·lis
trans·verse
trans·ver·sec·to·my
trans·ver·sus
trans·ves·tism
tra·pe·zi·um
tra·pe·zi·us
trap·e·zoid
trau·ma
trau·mat·ic
trau·ma·tism
trau·ma·ti·za·tion
trau·ma·top·a·thy
trau·ma·top·nea
tra·vail
treat·ment
tre·ma
trem·a·to·da

trem·a·tode
trem·bles
trem·bling
trem·el·loid
trem·or
trem·u·lant
trem·u·la·tion
trem·u·lous
trench mouth
trep·a·nize
tre·pan·ning
tre·phine
tre·phin·ing
treph·one
trep·i·dant
trep·i·da·tion
trepo·ne·ma
trep·o·ne·ma·to·sis
tri·ad
tri·age
tri·al
tri·an·gle
tri·an·gu·la·ris
tri·at·o·ma
tri·atom·ic
tri·ax·i·al
tri·ba·sic
tri·bas·i·lar
tri·bo·lu·mi·nes-
  cence
tri·bro·mo·eth·a-
  nol
tri·bu·ty·rin
tri·ceps
tri·chi·a·sis
trich·i·nel·li·a·sis

trich·i·no·sis
trich·i·on
trich·i·tis
trich·o·der·ma
trich·oid n.
tri·choid adj.
trich·o·lo·gia
tri·cho·ma
tri·cho·ma·de·sis
tri·cho·ma·to·sis
tri·chome
tri·cho·mic
trich·o·mon·as
trich·o·my·co·sis
trich·o·no·do·sis
trich·o·no·sis
trich·o·phy·ton
trich·o·phyt·o·sis
trich·or·rhea
trich·or·rhex·is
tri·cho·sis
trich·o·spo·ron
tri·chot·o·my
tri·chro·mat
tri·chro·mat·ic
tri·chro·mic
trich·u·ris
tri·cro·tism
tri·cro·tous
tri·cus·pid
tri·dac·tyl
tri·dent
tri·den·tate
tri·der·mic
trid·y·mus
tri·fid

tri·fo·cal
tri·fur·cate
tri·fur·ca·tion
tri·gas·tric
tri·gem·i·nal
tri·gem·i·nus
tri·gem·i·ny
tri·gen·ic
tri·gon
trig·o·nal
trig·o·nel·la
tri·go·nid
tri·go·ni·tis
trigo·no·no·ceph·a·lus
trigo·no·no·ceph·a·ly
tri·go·num
tri·labe
tri·lam·i·nar
tri·loc·u·lar
tri·loc·u·late
tri·men·su·al
tri·mes·ter
tri·o·nym
tri·or·chid
trip·a·ra
tri·pha·sic
tri·ple·gia
trip·let
tri·plex
trip·sis
tri·que·trum
tris·mus
tri·so·mus
tris·tis
trit·an·opia
tri·ti·ceous

tri·ti·um
tri·to·cone
tri·to·co·nid
trit·u·ra·ble
trit·u·rate
trit·u·ra·tion
tri·va·lence
tri·valve
tri·val·vu·lar
tro·car
tro·chan·ter
tro·che
tro·chis·ca·tion
tro·chis·cus
troch·lea
troch·le·ar
troch·o·ce·pha·lia
tro·choid
trom·bic·u·la
trom·bid·i·um
trom·o·ma·nia
tro·pe·sis
troph·e·sy
tro·phic
tropho·dy·nam·ics
tro·phol·o·gy
tropho·neu·ro·sis
troph·o·tax·is
trop·i·cal
tro·pism
tro·pom·e·ter
trun·cat·ed
trun·cus
truss
tryp·a·nide
try·pa·no·cide

try·pa·no·so·ma
try·pa·no·so·mi·a-
   sis
tryp·ars·amide
tryp·sin
tryp·sin·o·gen
tset·se
tu·ba
tub·age
tub·al
tu·bec·to·my
tu·ber
tu·ber·cle
tu·ber·cu·lar
tu·ber·cu·lat·ed
tu·ber·cu·la·tion
tu·ber·cu·lid or
   tu·ber·cu·lide
tu·ber·cu·lin
tu·ber·cu·lo·der·ma
tu·ber·cu·loid
tu·ber·cu·lo·ma
tu·ber·cu·lo·sis
tu·ber·cu·lous
tu·ber·cu·lum
tu·ber·os·i·ty
tu·bo·o·va·ri·an
tu·bo·u·ter·ine
tu·bo·vag·i·nal
tu·bu·lar
tu·bu·la·tion
tu·bule
tu·bu·lus
tu·bus
tug·ging
tu·la·re·mia

103

tu·me·fa·cient
tu·me·fac·tion
tu·me·fy
tu·men·tia
tu·mes·cence
tu·mes·cent
tu·mid
tu·mid·i·ty
tu·mor
tu·mor·al
tu·mor·ous
tu·mul·tus
tun·ga
tung·sten
tu·nic
tu·ni·ca
tun·nel
tur·bid
tur·bi·dim·e·ter
tur·bi·di·met·ric
tur·bi·di·met·ri·cal·ly
tur·bi·dim·e·try
tur·bid·i·ty
tur·bi·nate
tur·bi·nat·ed
tur·bi·nec·to·my
tur·ges·cence
tur·ges·cen·cy
tur·ges·cent
tur·gid
tur·gor
turn·ing
tur·pen·tine
tur·peth
tus·sal

tus·se·do
tus·sis
tus·sive
twang
tweez·ers
twi·light
twinge
twin·ning
twitch
twitch·ing
ty·lo·ma
ty·lo·sis
ty·lo·ste·re·sis
ty·lot·ic
tym·pa·nec·to·my
tym·pan·ic
tym·pa·nism
tym·pa·ni·tes
(distention of abdo-
men; cf. *tympanitis*)
tym·pa·nit·ic
tym·pa·ni·tis
(inflammation of ear
drum; cf. *tympanites*)
tym·pa·no·sis
tym·pa·not·o·my
tym·pa·nous
tym·pa·num
tym·pa·ny
typh·lec·ta·sia
typh·lec·to·my
typh·loid
typh·lo·sis
typh·lo·sole
ty·phoid
ty·phoi·dal

ty·phous adj.
ty·phus n.
typ·i·cal
typ·ing
ty·ra·mine
tyr·an·nism
ty·rem·e·sis
ty·rog·ly·phus
ty·roid
ty·ro·sine
ty·ro·thri·cin

uber·ous
uber·ty
ul·cer
ul·cer·ate
ul·cer·ation
ul·cer·ative
ul·cer·ous
ul·cus
ulet·ic
uli·tis
ul·na
ul·no·car·pe·us
uloc·a·ce
ulo·glos·si·tis
uloid
ulor·rha·gia

ulo·sis
ulot·ic
ulot·o·my
ul·ti·mo·gen·i·ture
ul·ti·mum·mor·i·ens
ul·tra·cen·tri·fuge
ul·tra·son·ic
um·ber
um·bi·lec·to·my
um·bil·i·cal
um·bil·i·cate
um·bil·i·cat·ed
um·bil·i·ca·tion
um·bi·li·cus
um·bo
un·cia sing.
un·ci·ae pl.
un·ci·nate
un·con·scious
un·con·scious·ness
unc·tion
unc·tu·ous
un·der·weight
un·dine
un·dine drop·per
un·do·ing
un·du·lant
un·du·la·tion
un·du·la·to·ry
un·gual
un·guen·tine
un·guen·tum
un·guis
uni·ar·tic·u·lar
uni·cam·er·al

uni·cel·lu·lar
uni·cen·tral
uni·cus·pid
uni·grav·i·da
uni·lat·er·al
uni·lo·bar
uni·loc·u·lar
uni·nu·cle·ar
uni·oc·u·lar
union
uni·ov·al
uni·ov·u·lar
unip·a·ra
unip·a·rous
uni·po·tent
uni·po·ten·cy
uni·po·ten·tial
uni·sex·u·al
uni·tary
uni·va·lent
un·of·fi·cial
un·or·ga·nized
un·rest
un·sat·u·rat·ed
un·sex
un·sound·ness
un·stri·at·ed
un·unit·ed
un·well
ura·cra·sia
ura·gogue
ura·ni·um
ura·no·plas·ty
ura·no·ple·gia
ura·nor·rha·phy
ura·nos·chi·sis

urate
ura·te·mia
ura·tu·ria
ur·ban·iza·tion
urea
ure·mia
ure·mic
ure·si·es·the·sia
ure·sis
ure·ter
ure·ter·al
ure·ter·ic
ure·ter·itis
ure·ter·o·cele
ure·ter·o·cys·tic
ure·ter·o·en·ter·ic
ure·ter·os·to·my
ure·ter·ot·o·my
ure·thra sing.
ure·thral
ure·thras or ure·thrae pl.
ure·thrit·i·des pl.
ure·thri·tis sing.
ure·thro·bulb·ar
ure·thro·cele
ure·thro·pro·stat·ic
ure·thro·scope
ure·thro·scop·ic
ure·thro·tome
ure·throt·o·my
ure·thro·vag·i·nal
ur·gen·cy
ur·hi·dro·sis
uric
uri·nal

105

uri·nal·y·sis
uri·nary
uri·nate
uri·na·tion
uri·na·tive
urine
uri·nif·ic
uri·nip·a·rous
uri·no·gen·i·tal
uri·nog·e·nous
uri·no·ma
uri·nom·e·ter
uri·no·scop·ic
uri·nose
uro·chrome
uro·clep·sia
uro·cris·ia
uro·cri·sis
uro·dae·um
uro·gen·i·tal
urog·e·nous
uro·glau·cin
uro·gram
urog·ra·phy
uro·ki·net·ic
uro·lith
uro·lith·ic
uro·li·thi·a·sis
uro·lith·ot·o·my
uro·log·ic
urol·o·gist
urol·o·gy
uro·lu·te·in
uron·on·com·e·try
uro·nos·co·py
urop·a·thy

uro·phan
uro·phan·ic
uro·phe·in
uror·rha·gia
uror·rho·din
uro·ru·bin
uros·cop·ic
uros·co·pist
uros·co·py
uro·se·in
uro·tox·ic
uro·tox·ic·i·ty
ur·ti·ca
ur·ti·car·ia
ur·ti·car·i·al
ur·ti·cate
ur·ti·ca·tion
uru·shi·ol
us·tion
uter·al·gia
uteri (sing.: *uterus*)
uter·ine
uter·is·mus
uter·i·tis
uter·o·cer·vi·cal
uter·o·col·ic
uter·o·ges·ta·tion
uter·o·in·tes·ti·nal
uter·o—o·va·ri·an
uter·o·pa·ri·e·tal
uter·o·pel·vic
uter·o·rec·tal
uter·o·sa·cral
uter·o·scope
uter·o·tub·al
uter·o·vag·i·nal

uter·o·ven·tral
uter·o·ves·i·cal
uter·us (pl.: *uteri*)
utri·cle
uvea
uve·itis
uvi·o·re·sist·ant
uvu·la sing.
uvu·lar
uvu·las or uvu-
lae pl.

vac·ci·na·ble
vac·ci·nal
vac·ci·nate
vac·ci·na·tion
vac·cine
vac·cin·i·o·la
vac·ci·noid
vac·u·o·lar
vac·u·o·late
vac·u·o·lat·ed
vac·u·o·la·tion
vac·u·ole
vac·u·um
va·gal
va·gi·na sing.

va·gi·nae *or* va-
gi·nas pl.
va·gi·nal
vag·i·nec·to·my
vag·i·nis·mus
vag·i·ni·tis
vag·i·no·fix·a·tion
vag·i·no·scope
vag·i·nos·co·py
vag·i·not·o·my
va·gi·tus
va·got·o·my
va·go·to·nia
va·go·ton·ic
va·grant
va·gus
va·lence
val·e·tu·di·nar·i·an
val·e·tu·di·nar·i-
an·ism
val·gus
val·late
val·lec·u·la sing.
val·lec·u·lae pl.
val·vot·o·my
val·vu·la sing.
val·vu·lae pl.
val·vu·lar
val·vu·li·tis
val·vu·lo·tome
val·vu·lot·o·my
vam·pire
va·nil·la
va·nil·lism
va·por
va·por·iza·tion

va·por·ize
va·por·iz·er
va·po·ther·a·py
vari·abil·i·ty
vari·able
vari·ance
vari·ant
vari·a·tion
var·i·ca·tion
var·i·cec·to·my
var·i·cel·la
var·i·cel·la·tion
var·i·ces (sing.: *varix*)
var·i·co·cele
var·i·cog·ra·phy
var·i·coid
var·i·co·phle·bi·tis
var·i·cose
var·i·co·sis
var·i·cos·i·ty
var·i·cot·o·my
va·ric·u·la
vari·ety
vari·form
va·ri·o·la
va·ri·o·lar
var·i·ol·ic
var·i·ol·i·form
va·ri·o·loid
var·ix (pl.: *varices*)
var·us
vas
vas·cu·lar·i·ty
vas·cu·lar·iza·tion
vas   de·fer·ens

va·sec·to·my
Vas·e·line
vas·i·fac·tion
vas·i·tis
va·so·con·stric·tion
va·so·con·stric·tive
va·so·de·pres·sor
va·so·di·la·ta·tion
or
va·so·di·la·tion
va·so·dil·a·tin
va·so·di·la·tor
va·sog·ra·phy
va·so·in·hib·i·tor
vas·o·li·ga·tion
vas·o·punc·ture
vas·or·rha·phy
vas·o·sec·tion
vas·os·to·my
vas·ot·o·my
vas·o·ton·ic
va·so·va·gal
vas·tus
vec·tion
vec·tis
vec·tor
vec·to·ri·al
veg·e·ta·tion
ve·hi·cle
vein
ve·la (sing.: *velum*)
ve·la·men sing.
ve·lam·i·na pl.
vel·li·cate
vel·li·ca·tion
ve·lum (pl.: *vela*)

ve·na sing.
ve·nae pl.
ve·na·tion
ven·ec·to·my
ven·e·nif·er·ous
ve·ne·re·al
ve·ne·re·ol·o·gist
ve·ne·re·ol·o·gy *or*
  ven·er·ol·o·gy
ve·ne·re·o·pho·bia
ven·ery
vene·sec·tion *or*
  veni·sec·tion
ven·e·su·ture
veni·punc·ture
veno·cly·sis
veno·gram
ve·nog·ra·phy
ven·om·ous
ve·no·scle·ro·sis
ve·nos·i·ty
ve·no·sta·sis
ve·no·throm·bot·ic
ve·not·o·my
ve·nous
vent
ven·ter
ven·ti·late
ven·ti·la·tion
ven·tral
ven·tri·cle
ven·tric·u·lar
ven·tric·u·li·tes
ven·tric·u·lo·gram
ven·tric·u·log·ra-
  phy

ven·tric·u·lus
ven·tri·cum·bent
ven·tri·duc·tion
ven·tri·me·sal
ven·tro·me·di·an
ven·tros·co·py
ven·trose
ven·tros·i·ty
ven·ule
ver·big·er·a·tion
ver·gen·ces
ver·gens
ver·mes (sing.:
  vermis)
ver·mic·u·lose
ver·mi·fuge
ver·min
ver·mi·na·tion
ver·mis (pl.: *vermes*)
ver·ru·ca
ver·ru·ci·form
ver·ru·coid
ver·ru·cose
ver·si·col·ored
ver·te·bra sing.
ver·te·brae *or*
  ver·te·bras pl.
ver·te·brate
ver·te·brec·to·my
ver·tex
ver·ti·cal
ver·ti·cil
ver·ti·cil·late
ver·tig·i·nous
ver·ti·go
ve·si·ca

ves·i·cal
ves·i·ca·tion
ves·i·cle (small sac
  of fluid; cf. *visical*)
ves·i·cot·o·my
ves·i·co·u·ter·ine
ve·sic·u·la
ve·sic·u·lar
ve·sic·u·la·tion
ve·sic·u·lec·to·my
ve·sic·u·li·tis
ve·sic·u·lo·bul·lous
ves·sel
ves·ti·bule
ves·tige
ve·ta
vet·er·i·nar·i·an
vet·er·i·nary
vi·a·ble
vi·al (container)
vi·bra·tion
vi·bra·tor
vi·bris·sa sing.
vi·bris·sae pl.
vi·car·i·ous
vid·e·og·no·sis
vig·il·am·bu·lism
vig·i·lance
vil·lous adj.
vil·lus n.
vin·cu·lum
vin·e·gar
vi·nyl
vi·o·la·tion
vi·o·let
vi·o·my·cin

vi·re·mia
vir·gin·i·ty
vir·ile
vir·i·les·cence
vir·il·ism
vir·i·lis·mus
vi·ril·i·ty
vi·rip·o·tent
vi·rol·o·gist
vi·rol·o·gy
vir·u·lence
vir·u·len·cy
vir·u·lif·er·ous
vi·rus
vis *or* viss
vis·cera (sing.: *viscus*)
vis·cer·al
vis·cer·al·gia
vis·cid
vis·cos·i·ty
vis·cous adj.
vis·cus (pl.: *viscera*)
vis·i·bil·i·ty
vis·i·ble
vis·i·cal adj.
  (pertaining to urinary
  bladder; cf. *vesicle*)
vi·sion
vi·su·al·iza·tion
vis·u·o·sen·so·ry
vi·sus
vi·ta·gen
vi·tal·i·ty
vi·ta·min
vi·tel·lus
vit·i·li·go

vit·i·li·goid
vit·re·ous
vi·tres·cence
vit·ric
vi·tri·na
vit·ri·tis
vit·rum
viv·i·fi·ca·tion
vi·vip·a·rous
vivi·sec·tion
vo·cal
vo·ca·lis
vola
vol·a·tile
vol·a·til·iza·tion
vol·a·til·ize
vo·le·mic
vo·li·tion
volt·age
vol·ta·me·ter
volt·me·ter
vol·ume
vol·un·tary
vo·mer
vom·it·ing
vom·i·tive
vom·i·to·ry
vom·i·tu·ri·tion
vom·i·tus
vo·ra·cious
vor·tex
vor·ti·cose
vox
vul·ner·a·ble
vul·va
vul·vi·tis

wad·ding
wad·dle
wa·fer
waist
wake·ful·ness
wan·der·ing
wart
watt·age
wean
weep·ing
weight
welt
wen
wheal
wheeze
whey
whiff
whis·per
whoop
whoop·ing   cough
win·dow
wind·pipe
wink
wir·ing
wiry
with·draw·al
womb
wrin·kles
wrist
wry·neck

xan·tho·ma sing.
xan·tho·mas *or*
  xan·tho·ma·ta pl.
xan·tho·sis
xan·thous
xan·thox·y·lum
xen·o·me·nia
xeno·pho·bia
xen·oph·thal·mia
xen·o·pus
xe·ran·tic
xe·ro·der·ma
xe·ro·myc·te·ria
xer·on·o·sus
xe·roph·thal·mia
xe·ro·ses pl.
xe·ro·sis sing
xe·ro·sto·mia
xe·ro·tes
xe·rot·ic
xe·ro·trip·sis
xiph·oid·i·tis
X   ray n.
X-ray v., adj.

yaw·ey
yawn·ing
yaws
yeast
yel·low
yo·gurt *or* yo-
  ghurt
yolk
youth

Z

zar·an·than
ze·ro
zinc
zo·na sing.
zo·nae *or* zo·nas
  pl.

zon·al
zone
zon·es·the·sia
zo·nif·u·gal
zo·nip·e·tal
zo·nu·lar
zo·nule
zo·o·der·mic
zo·ol·o·gist
zoo·no·sis
zoo·par·a·site
zos·ter·i·form
zos·ter·oid
zwie·back
zy·go·ma
zy·go·mat·ic
zy·go·mat·i-
  cus
zy·go·spore
zy·go·style
zy·gote
zy·go·tene
zy·got·ic
zyl·caine
zy·mase
zyme
zy·mo·gen·ic
zy·moid
zy·mol·o·gy
zy·mo·ne·ma

Reference Section

Variations in the use of periods and capitalization with medical abbreviations are widespread.

Abbreviation	Meaning
A_1	Aortic first sound
A_2	Aortic second sound
$A_2 = P_2$	Aortic second sound equals pulmonic second sound
$A_2 > P_2$	Aortic second sound is greater than pulmonic second sound
$A_2 < P_2$	Aortic second sound is less than pulmonic second sound
A.A.	Achievement age; Alcoholics Anonymous
$\overline{AA}$, $\overline{aa}$	Of each
aa	Equal parts of each
abdom.	Abdomen
a.c.	Before meals (*ante cibum*)
ACC	Anodal closure contraction
Acc.	Accommodation
A.C.D.	Absolute cardiac dullness
ACE	Adrenocortical extract
ACTH	Adrenocorticolropic hormone
A.D.	Right ear (*auris dextra*)
ad; admov	Add; let there be added
ad lib	At pleasure; as much as needed
Adv.	Against
A-G	Albumin-globulin ratio

Alt. dieb.	Every other day
Alt. hor.	Every other hour
alt. noct.	Every other night
A.P.	Anterior pituitary; axiopupal; antero-posterior
a.p.	Before dinner (*ante prandium*)
Aq.	Water
Aq. dest.	Distilled water
ARD.	Acute respiratory disease
As.	Astigmatism; arsenic
A.S.	Left ear
A.V.	Atrioventricular; arteriovenous
Av.	Average; avoirdupois
AZT.	Aschheim-Zondek test
BBT.	Basal body temperature
b.d.	Twice a day
BFP.	Biologic false positive reaction
Bib.	Drink
b.i.d.	Twice a day (*bis in die*)
B.M.	Seawater bath; bowel movement
B.M.R.	Basal metabolic rate
B.P.	Blood pressure
b.p.	Boiling point
b.r.p.	Bathroom privileges
B.S.	Breath sounds; blood sugar
B.T.U., B.Th.U.	British thermal unit
BUN.	Blood urea nitrogen
B.V.	Vapor bath
C.	Centigrade; cathode; carbon
C	Precordial lead (electrocardiogram)
CA.	Chronological age

Ca.	Calcium; cathode; carcinoma
Cath.	Cathartic
c.b.c.	Complete blood count
C.C.	Chief complaint
cc.	Cubic centimeter
cf.	Compare; bring together
Cg.; Cgm.	Centigram
C.m.	Tomorrow morning
cm.	Centimeter
cm.^{3}	Cubic centimeter
c.mm.	Cubic millimeter
C.M.R.	Cerebral metabolic rate
c.m.s.	To be taken tomorrow morning
C.n.	Tomorrow night
C.N.S.	Central nervous system
c.n.s.	To be taken tomorrow night
Collut.	Mouthwash
Collyr.	Eyewash
Cont. rem.	Let the medicine be continued
Coq.	Boil
c.p.m.	Counts per minute
C.S.	Current strength
Cs.	Conscious; consciousness
C.S.F.	Cerebrospinal fluid
C.S.M.	Cerebrospinal meningitis
CST.	Convulsive shock therapy
cu. mm	Cubic millimeter
c.v.	Tomorrow evening (*cras vespere*)
C.V.A.	Costrovertebral angle
Cx.	Convex
D.	Dose; distal; dorsal; duration

D. & C.	Dilation and curettement
D-1 to D-12	Dorsal vertebra (1 to 12)
D.A.H.	Disordered action of heart
D.D.S.	Doctor of Dental Surgery
DDT	Chlorophenothane
Decub.	Lying down
de d. in d.	From day to day
Deg.	Degeneration; degree
dg.	Decigram
Dieb. alt.	On alternate days
Dieb. tert	Every third day
dil.	Dilute; dissolve
dim.	One half
Dir. prop.	With proper direction
DMF.	Accumulated dental caries
D.O.A.	Dead on arrival
D.O.B.	Date of birth
D.P.	Pulses (*dorsalis pedis*)
dr.	Dram
D.T.	Distance test
D.T.D.	Give of such a dose
D.T.P.	Distal tingling on percussion
DTR's	Deep tendon reflexes
D.V.M.	Doctor of Veterinary Medicine
E.C.T.	Electric convulsive therapy
E.D.	Effective dose
EEG	Electroencephalogram
EENT	Ears, eyes, nose, and throat
e.g.	For example (*exempli gratis*)
E.j.	Elbow jerk
EKG	Electrocardiogram

EKY	Electrokymogram
EMG	Electromyogram
emul.	Emulsion
E.N.T	Ear, nose, and throat
E.O.M.	Extraocular movements
EPR	Electrophrenic respiration
E.R.	External resistance
ERG	Electroretinogram
ESP	Extrasensory perception
E.S.T.	Electroshock therapy
F.	Fahrenheit; field of vision; formula
F & R	Force and rhythm
FB	Fingerbreadth
FBS	Fasting blood sugar
F.D.	Focal distance; fatal dose
F.D.A.; F.D.P.; F.D.T.	Positions of the fetus
Feb. dur.	While the fever lasts
F.F.A.	Free fatty acids
F.H.	Family history
fl.; fld.	Fluid
F.L.A.; F.L.P.; F.L.T.	Positions of the fetus
F.M.	Make a mixture
F.U.O.	Fever of undetermined origin
G.; g.; gm.	Gram
G.B.	Gallbladder
G.I.	Gastrointestinal; globin insulin
gl.	Gland
G.P.	General practitioner
gr.	Grain
G.S.W.	Gunshot wound
gt.; gtt.	Drop

g.u.	Genitourinary
H.	Hydrogen; hour
Hb.	Hemoglobin
HCT.	Hematocrit
H.D.	Hearing distance
H.d.	At bedtime
H.D.L.W.	Distance watch is heard by left ear
H.D.R.W	Distance watch is heard by right ear
H.E.D.	Unit of roentgen-ray dosage
Hg.; Hgb	Hemoglobin
H_2O	Water
Hor. decub.	At bedtime
Hor. interm.	At the intermediate hours
hpf	High-power field
H.S.	House surgeon
h.s.	At bedtime
ht.	Height
IC	Inspiratory capacity
ID	Inside diameter; infective dose
Id.	Same
I.H.	Infectious hepatitus
I.M.	Intramuscularly
in.	Inch
in d.	Daily
IOP	Intraocular pressure
I.Q.	Intelligence quotient
I.R.	Internal resistance
I.S.	Intercostal space
I.V.	Intravenously
I.V.T.	Intravenous transfusion
k.	Constant

kg.	Kilogram
kg.-m.	Kilogram-meter
k.k.	Knee kicks (knee jerks)
K.U.B.	Kidney, ureter, and bladder
kv.	Kilovolt
kvp.	Kilovolt peak
kw.	Kilowatt
kw.-hr.	Kilowatt-hour
L.	Liter; lumbar
L. and A.	Light and accommodation
lb.	Pound
L.E.	Left eye
L.F.A.; L.F.P.; L.F.T.	Positions of the fetus
L.L.L.	Left lower lobe (lungs)
L.M.A.; L.M.P.; L.M.T.	Positions of the fetus
L.M.P.	Last menstrual period
L.O.A.; L.O.P.; L.O.T.	Positions of the fetus
L.P.	Lumbar puncture; linguopulpal
lpf.	Low power field
L.S.D.	Hallucinogenic
L.S.A.; L.S.P.; L.S.T.	Positions of the fetus
L.U.L.	Left upper lobe (lungs)
M.	Meter; mixture; muscle
m.	Meter
M.A.	Mental age
ma.	Milliampere
m.b.	Mix well
mc.	Millicurie
mcg.	Microgram
MCV	Mean corpuscular volume
M.D.	Doctor of Medicine

M.D.A.; M.D.P.; M.D.T.	Positions of the fetus
M.E.D.	Minimal effective dose
mEq.	Milliequivalent
M. et sig.	Mix and write a label
mg.	Milligram
M.I.D.	Minimum infective dose
ml.	Milliliter
M.M.	Mucous membranes
mM.	Millimole
mm.	Millimeter; muscles
Mol. wt.	Molecular weight
mp.	Melting point
mr.	Milliroentgen
M.S.L.	Midsternal line
M.V.	Veterinary physician
mv.	Millivolt
My.	Myopia
N.A.D.	No appreciable disease
nn.	Nerves
N.N.D.	New and nonofficial drugs
Noct. maneq.	At night and in the morning
N.T.P.	Normal temperature and pressure
Nv.	Naked vision
N.Y.D.	Not yet diagnosed
O.	Oxygen; eye
OB	Obstetrics
O.D.	Right eye; outside diameter
O.D.A.; O.D.P.; O.D.T.	Positions of the fetus
O.L.	Left eye
O.L.A.; O.L.P.; O.L.T.	Positions of the fetus
o.m.	Every morning

Omn. bih.	Every two hours
Omn. noct.	Every night
o.n.	Every night
OPD	Outpatient department
o.s.	Left eye
OTD	Organ tolerance radiation dose
O.U.	Both eyes
Ov.	Egg
oz.	Ounce
P.	Pulse; pupil
P_2	Pulmonic second sound
P & A	Percussion and auscultation
P.A.	Pulpo-axial
P. ae.	In equal parts
Part. aeq.	Equal parts
Part. vic.	In divided doses
P.C.	Avoirdupois weight
p.c.	After meals
pcpt.	Perception
Pcs.	Preconscious
P.E.	Physical examination
P.E.G.	Pneumoencephalography
P.H.	Past history
pH	Hydrogen ion concentration
P.L.	Light perception
P.M.I.	Point of maximal impulse
P.N.	Percussion note
P.O.	By mouth; orally
P. rat. aetat.	In proportion to age
p.r.n.	According as circumstances may require

p.s.	Per second
p.s.i.	Pounds per square inch
P.S.P.	Phenolsulfonphthalein
pt.	Pint
PTA; PTC	Blood coagulation factors
Px.	Pneumothorax
q.d.	Every day
q.h.	Every hour
q.i.d.	Four times a day
q.l.	As much as desired
q.p.	At will
q.q.h.	Every four hours
q.s.	Sufficient quantity
q. suff.	As much as suffices
qt.	Quart
q.v.	As much as you please
R.	Respiration; roentgen
℞	Take
rbc.	Red blood cell; red blood count
R.E.	Right eye
R.E.G.	Radioencephalogram
Reg. umb.	Umbilical region
Rep.	Repeat
R.F.A.; R.F.P.; R.F.T.	Positions of the fetus
R.L.L.	Right lower lobe (lungs)
R.M.	Respiratory movement
R.M.A.; R.M.P.; R.M.T.	Positions of the fetus
R.M.L.	Right middle lobe (lungs)
R.N.	Registered Nurse
R.O.A.; R.O.P.; R.O.T.	Positions of the fetus
rpm	Revolutions per minute

R.Q.	Respiratory quotient
R.S.A.; R.S.P.; R.S.T.	Positions of the fetus
R.T.	Reading test
R.U.L.	Right upper lobe (lung)
S.	Sacral; sulfur
s.c.	Subcutaneously
S.D.A.; S.D.P.; S.D.T.	Positions of the fetus
S.E.	Standard error
Sed.	Stool
Seq. luce.	The following day
S.I.	Soluble insulin
Si op. sit.	If it is necessary
S.L.A.; S.L.P.; S.L.T.	Positions of the fetus
S.N.	According to nature
S.O.S.	If it is necessary
sp. gr.	Specific gravity
SQ	Subcutaneous
S.R.	Sedimentation rate
ss.	One half
s.s.	Soapsuds
S.T.S.	Serologic test for syphilis
su.	Let him take
s.v.	Alcoholic spirit
T.	Temperature; thoracic
t.	Temporal
T.A.; T.A.T.	Toxin-antitoxin
TB	Tuberculosis
T.b.	Tubercle bacillus
t.d.s.	Three times a day
Te.	Tetanus
t.i.d.	Three times a day

TLC	Tender loving care; total lung capacity
tr.	Tincture
T.S.	Test solution
T.U.	Toxic unit
TV	Tuberculin volutin
U.	Unit
U.S.P., U. S. Phar.	United States Pharmacopeia
Ut dict.	As directed
Utend.	To be used
V.	Vision
v.	Vein; volt
Va.	Visual acuity
V. & T.	Volume and tension (pulse)
V.C.	Acuity of color vision
V.D.	Venereal disease
V.D.G.	Venereal disease—gonorrhea
V.D.S.	Venereal disease—syphilis
Ves.	Bladder
V.F.	Vocal fremitus
V.f.	Field of vision
V.M.	Voltmeter
v.s.	Vibration seconds
vv.	Veins
V.W.	Vessel wall
wbc.	White blood cell; white blood cell count
W.R.	Wassermann reaction
Wt.	Weight
X.	Unit of x-ray dosage
z.	Symbol for atomic number
Z.Z.'Z."	Increasing degrees of contraction